AF838832

Biomedical Materials for Multi-functional Applications

Series Editors

Arnab Chanda, Centre for Biomedical Engineering, Indian Institute of Technology Delhi, New Delhi, India

Sarabjeet Sidhu, Department of Mechanical Engineering, Sardar Beant Singh State University, Gurdaspur, India

The series 'Biomedical Materials for Multi-functional Applications' is intended for the audience with an interest in biomaterials for various applications, including bio-implants, bio-instrumentation, biomechanics, and tissue engineering. The book titles under this series will bring different areas of biomedical engineering, bioengineering, materials science, mechanical engineering, and biosciences under one umbrella of biomedical materials. The books in this series will provide deep insights into the state-of-art of biomedical materials and deal with diverse and interdisciplinary aspects of biomaterials, ranging from basic science to host responses, as well as real-time applications. Some of the topics include but are not limited to: functional materials, smart materials, biomimetic materials, polymers, composites, ceramics, metals, alloys, and nanomaterials. This series will provide the most recent advances in biomedical materials, including design, synthesis, processing, and characterization. This series will accept both authored and edited volumes, including monographs, textbooks, reference works, and handbooks. This series aims to publish new advances in biomedical materials that have been made in the fabrication and development of biomaterials for different applications and the advancement of principles, theories, and designs. Each book title in the series will give a comprehensive overview of pioneering topics, and the readers will gain new knowledge and insights about the topic. As a collection, the series on 'Biomedical Materials for Multi-functional Applications' is anticipated to benefit a wide audience in academia, the research community, and industry.

Amit Mahajan · Sandeep Devgan · Gurpreet Singh

Surface Modification of Co–Cr Alloy for Orthopaedic Applications

Springer

Amit Mahajan
Department of Mechanical Engineering
Khalsa College of Engineering
and Technology
Amritsar, Punjab, India

Sandeep Devgan
Department of Mechanical Engineering
Khalsa College of Engineering
and Technology
Amritsar, Punjab, India

Gurpreet Singh
Centre for Biomedical Engineering
Indian Institute of Technology Delhi
New Delhi, Delhi, India

ISSN 2731-9695 ISSN 2731-9709 (electronic)
Biomedical Materials for Multi-functional Applications
ISBN 978-981-95-4028-0 ISBN 978-981-95-4029-7 (eBook)
https://doi.org/10.1007/978-981-95-4029-7

© The Editor(s) (if applicable) and The Author(s), under exclusive license to Springer Nature Singapore Pte Ltd. 2026

This work is subject to copyright. All rights are solely and exclusively licensed by the Publisher, whether the whole or part of the material is concerned, specifically the rights of translation, reprinting, reuse of illustrations, recitation, broadcasting, reproduction on microfilms or in any other physical way, and transmission or information storage and retrieval, electronic adaptation, computer software, or by similar or dissimilar methodology now known or hereafter developed.
The use of general descriptive names, registered names, trademarks, service marks, etc. in this publication does not imply, even in the absence of a specific statement, that such names are exempt from the relevant protective laws and regulations and therefore free for general use.
The publisher, the authors and the editors are safe to assume that the advice and information in this book are believed to be true and accurate at the date of publication. Neither the publisher nor the authors or the editors give a warranty, expressed or implied, with respect to the material contained herein or for any errors or omissions that may have been made. The publisher remains neutral with regard to jurisdictional claims in published maps and institutional affiliations.

This Springer imprint is published by the registered company Springer Nature Singapore Pte Ltd.
The registered company address is: 152 Beach Road, #21-01/04 Gateway East, Singapore 189721, Singapore

If disposing of this product, please recycle the paper.

Preface

Orthopedic implants have transformed the quality of life for millions of individuals suffering from joint degeneration, bone fractures, and skeletal deformities. Among the various materials employed in implant fabrication, cobalt-chromium (Co–Cr) alloys have stood out due to their exceptional mechanical strength, corrosion resistance, and long-term stability in the human body. However, despite their durability, Co–Cr alloys often exhibit limited bioactivity, which can impede osseointegration and long-term biological performance. The clinical need to overcome these limitations motivated the present work, which is focused on surface modification strategies to enhance the biological and mechanical performance of Co–Cr alloys for orthopedic applications. This monograph is the result of an extensive research effort combining material science, biomedical engineering, and surface engineering to develop a novel electro-discharge coating approach for Co–Cr alloys. The work is structured into eight chapters, each building upon the previous to provide a detailed and coherent exploration of the topic. Beginning with an introduction to orthopedic implants and biomaterials, the book progresses through a comprehensive literature review, the rationale for surface modifications, and the selection of suitable materials. It then delves into the detailed methodology of electrical discharge machining (EDM) used for surface coating, followed by a systematic presentation of surface characterization techniques and experimental results. The concluding chapter synthesizes the findings and discusses the future prospects and potential applications of this research. The core of this monograph lies in its experimental and analytical rigor, supported by advanced characterization techniques including scanning electron microscopy (SEM), energy-dispersive spectroscopy (EDS), and X-ray diffraction (XRD), along with corrosion, wear, cytotoxicity, and hemolysis testing. These investigations not only confirmed the effectiveness of EDM-based coatings in improving surface bioactivity and mechanical properties but also opened new avenues for implant surface design tailored to specific clinical needs.

This monograph is intended for graduate students, researchers, and professionals working in the fields of biomaterials, surface engineering, and orthopedic implant development. It will also serve as a reference for interdisciplinary researchers exploring the interface of materials science and biomedical engineering. The content reflects the current challenges and advancements in the design of biocompatible surfaces for metallic implants and proposes a scalable, efficient, and adaptable approach through electro-discharge surface coating.

We hope this work contributes meaningfully to the ongoing efforts to design safer, smarter, and more effective orthopedic implants, ultimately benefiting both researchers and patients in the field of orthopedic healthcare.

Amritsar, Punjab, India Amit Mahajan
Amritsar, Punjab, India Sandeep Devgan
New Delhi, India Gurpreet Singh

Competing Interests The authors have no competing interests to declare that are relevant to the content of this manuscript.

Contents

1 Biomaterials for Medical Implants 1
1.1 Biomaterials Overview 1
1.2 Properties of Biomaterials 2
1.2.1 Physical Properties 2
1.2.2 Chemical Properties 4
1.2.3 Mechanical Properties 6
1.2.4 Biological Properties 7
1.3 Types of Biomaterials 9
References 15

2 Surface Engineering of Metallic Biomaterials 19
2.1 Stainless Steel 19
2.2 Magnesium 25
2.3 Titanium 28
2.4 Cobalt-Chromium 31
2.5 Conclusions 37
References 38

3 Electrical Discharge Machining for Surface Engineering of Biomedical Alloys 43
3.1 Principles of Electro Discharge Machining (EDM) 44
3.2 Background of EDM 45
3.3 Surface Engineering by EDM 47
3.3.1 Influence of EDM Parameters on Surface Modification 48
3.4 Biomedical Applications of Conventional EDM-Treated Surfaces 51
3.5 Applications of Powder-Mixed EDM in Biomedical Surface Engineering 54
3.6 Discussion and Overall Summary 61
3.7 Conclusions and Future Scope 62
References 63

4 Electric Discharge Treatment of Co–Cr Alloy 69
4.1 Experimental Framework 70
4.2 Workpiece Material: ASTM F75 Co–Cr Alloy 70
4.3 Variants Electrode Tool Employed for Experimental Work 74
4.4 Stage I: Full Factorial Design for Surface Roughness and Biocompatibility 75
4.5 Stage II: Multi-parameter Optimization Using Taguchi Design 77
4.6 Stage III: Validation of Optimized Conditions 78
4.7 Statistical Analysis 80
4.8 Advanced Characterization Techniques 80
4.9 Conclusions 81
References 82

5 In-Vitro Biocompatibility Analysis of EDMed Co–Cr Alloy (Stage I) 83
5.1 Description of Stage I Experimentation 83
5.1.1 Surface Roughness Evaluation 84
5.1.2 Evaluation of Biological Response of EDMed Surface 84
5.2 Results and Discussion 89
5.2.1 Surface Roughness 90
5.2.2 In-Vitro Biocompatibility Test 93
5.2.3 XRD Analysis 97
5.3 Conclusions 99
References 101

6 In-Vitro Corrosion Investigation of Co–Cr Alloy (Stage II) 103
6.1 Description of Stage II Experimentation 103
6.1.1 Electrochemical Corrosion Measurements 104
6.1.2 In-Vitro Hemolysis Test 106
6.2 Results and Discussion 107
6.2.1 Statistical Analysis 109
6.2.2 Electrochemical Corrosion Analysis 110
6.2.3 Hemocompatibility Analysis 114
6.2.4 XRD Analysis 115
6.3 Conclusions 118
References 119

7 Tribological Performance Analysis of Co–Cr Alloy (Stage III) 121
7.1 Selection of Parameters for Experimentation of Stage III 122
7.1.1 Pin-On-Disk Wear Study 123
7.1.2 In-Vitro Cytocompatibility Test 125
7.2 Results and Discussion 127
7.2.1 Cytocompatibility Analysis 127
7.2.2 Tribological Examination of EDMed Surfaces 129
7.2.3 EDX and XRD Analysis 134

7.3 Discussion ... 136
7.4 Conclusions ... 137
References ... 138

8 Conclusions and Future Scope ... 141
8.1 Summary of Key Findings ... 142
8.2 Future Research Directions ... 144
References ... 146

About the Authors

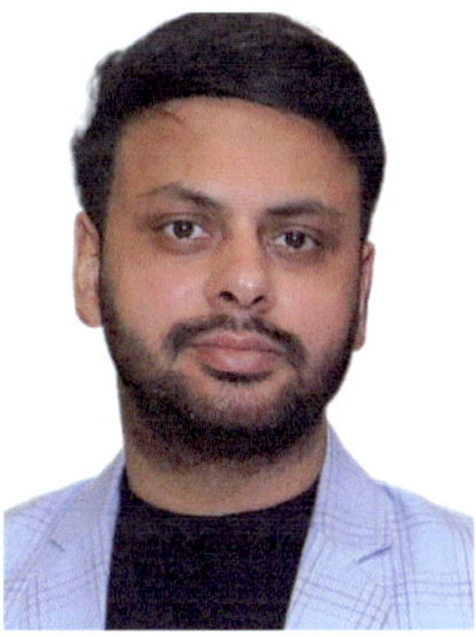

Dr. Amit Mahajan is an associate professor at Khalsa College of Engineering and Technology, Amritsar, India. His research interests include additive manufacturing, surface modification of biomaterials, and electrical discharge machining. He earned his Ph.D. in Mechanical Engineering from I. K. Gujral Punjab Technical University, Punjab, India, with his research interests in additive manufacturing, surface coating, bio-implants, and non-conventional machining. Currently, he works on the fabrication of alloys with a proper fraction composition of carbon nanotubes (CNTs) and μ-hydroxyapatite (μ-HAp) via additive manufacturing. He has contributed multiple research papers and chapters to international journals, books, and conferences. He has also edited a Springer book and conference proceedings. He has received several recognitions, including the Best Researcher Award (2020) from the Khalsa Society, the ISTE Best Teacher Award (2020), and the ISTE Best Researcher Award (2015). He also contributes as a reviewer for several international journals.

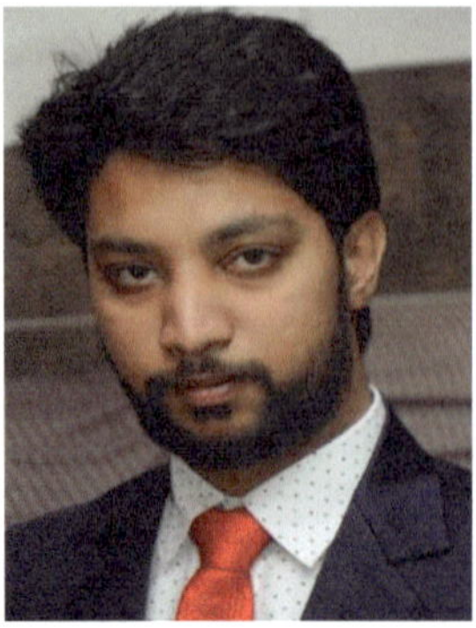

Dr. Sandeep Devgan is an associate professor at Khalsa College of Engineering and Technology, Amritsar, India. He earned his Ph.D. in Mechanical Engineering from I. K. Gujral Punjab Technical University, Punjab, India. His research interests include CNTs-based nanotechnology, surface modification of biomaterials, and powder-mixed electrical discharge machining. Currently, he works on alloy fabrication with the proper fraction composition of carbon nanotubes (CNTs) and μ-hydroxyapatite (μ-HAp) via additive manufacturing. He has contributed multiple research papers and chapters to international journals, books, and conferences. He has also edited a Springer book. He has received the ISTE Best Teacher Award (2022) and the ISTE Best Researcher Award (2015). He also currently serves as a reviewer for leading international journals.

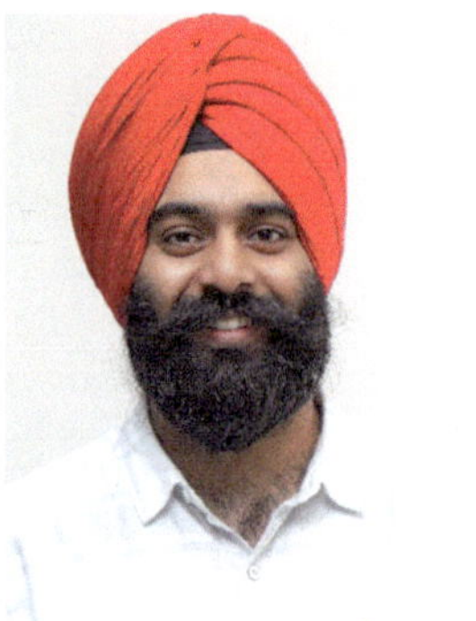

Dr. Gurpreet Singh is currently an Early-Doc Fellow at the Indian Institute of Technology (IIT) Delhi, where he earned his Ph.D. in Biomedical Engineering as a Prime Minister's Research Fellow (PMRF). His interdisciplinary research spans biomimetics, soft tissue mechanics, artificial tissue development, computational biomechanics, and medical intervention design. During his Ph.D., he developed biomechanical models for diabetic foot ulcers and designed a modular insole for pressure offloading. He has also worked on developing artificial tissue surrogates and computational models of brain aneurysms, integrating experimental and simulation approaches. Previously, he worked on surface modification of metallic biomaterials using electro-discharge machining to enhance bioactivity. He has contributed multiple peer-reviewed publications and book chapters in international journals and conferences. He has also authored some monograph books and co-edited a volume. He has received several recognitions, including the Top Cited Paper Award (IOP Publishing 2023) for his review article on the mechanical properties of soft human tissues, the Research Excellence Travel Award (RETA) from IIT Delhi in 2024, the Dogra Educational Endowment Award (2025), and a nomination for the Amit Garg Memorial Research Excellence Award. He is serving as a reviewer for leading international journals.

Abbreviations

ALD	Atomic Layer Deposition
AM	Additive Manufacturing
ANOVA	Analysis of Variance
ASTM	American Society for Testing and Materials
CNC	Computer Numerical Control
CNTs	Carbon Nanotubes
Co–Cr	Cobalt–Chromium
CR	Corrosion Rate
CVD	Chemical Vapor Deposition
DSS	Duplex Stainless Steel
EDC	Electrical Discharge Coating
EDM	Electrical Discharge Machining
EDS	Energy-Dispersive Spectroscopy
EDT	Electrical (or electro) Discharge Treatment
EDX	Energy Dispersive X-Ray Spectroscopy
FBS	Fetal Bovine Serum
FESEM	Field Emission Scanning Electron Microscopy
HAp	Hydroxyapatite
MWCNTs	Multi-Walled Carbon Nanotubes
PEO	Plasma Electrolytic Oxidation
PMEDM	Powder-Mixed EDM
PVD	Physical Vapor Deposition
RBCs	Red Blood Cells
RC	Resistance-Capacitance
SBF	Simulated Body Fluid
SD	Standard Deviation
SEM	Scanning Electron Microscopy
SiC	Silicon Carbide
W–Cu	Tungsten–Copper
XRD	X-Ray Diffraction

Symbols

mm^3	Cubic millimeter
A	Ampere
μm	Micrometer
μs	Microseconds
μV	Microvolt
mV	Millivolt
A/cm^2	Ampere per square centimeter
g/cm^3	Gram per cubic centimeter
V	Volt
kPa	Kilopascal
MPa	Megapascal
GPa	Gigapascal
Mm	Millimeter
mm/s	Millimeter per second
J	Joule
Hz	Hertz
L	Liter
HRC	Rockwell Hardness C scale
°C	Degree Celsius
N	Newton
rpm	Revolutions per minute
m/s	Meter per second
mg	Milligram
V	Voltage
S/N ratio	Signal-to-noise ratio
Ra	Average roughness
Ag/AgCl	Silver/silver chloride
E_{corr}	Corrosion potential
I_{corr}	Corrosion current density

Chapter 1
Biomaterials for Medical Implants

1.1 Biomaterials Overview

In contemporary medical practice, there is an increasing reliance on biomaterials across a wide array of applications, including tissue engineering, drug delivery systems, and advanced medical imaging techniques. These materials are meticulously designed to exhibit enhanced stability and optimized pharmacokinetic profiles to promote effective cellular growth and regeneration [1]. Biomaterials can be either synthetic or bioengineered, and they are introduced into living organisms to replace, support, or enhance biological structures and functions, often with the intention of long-term or even lifetime use [2]. Given their critical role in medical interventions, these materials must possess several key properties: they should be non-toxic, non-carcinogenic, chemically inert, structurally stable, and mechanically robust enough to withstand the ongoing physiological stresses encountered in a living environment [3]. In recent decades, the demand for and development of bioimplants has surged, driven by an aging population, increased life expectancy, shifting lifestyle patterns, and continuous innovations in implant technologies. Research has consistently demonstrated that the surface characteristics and microstructural features of biomaterials are crucial determinants in how these materials interact with biological tissues, significantly influencing biocompatibility and the success of osseointegration processes. Osseointegration, the process by which implants anchor to bone, is essential for the longevity and efficacy of various surgical implants [4]. The twenty-first century has witnessed a remarkable evolution in biomaterials, marked by a multidisciplinary approach that integrates therapeutic sciences, materials engineering, biochemistry, biomedical technologies, and clinical research. While the exploration of structural design, synthesis, manufacturing processes, and the physical properties of biomaterials is primarily rooted in materials science and engineering, the investigation of their biological behaviors and biochemical interactions falls under the domain of biochemistry [5]. Simultaneously, the field of biomedical science is critical in understanding how biomaterials engage with biological tissues, including

© The Author(s), under exclusive license to Springer Nature Singapore Pte Ltd. 2026

A. Mahajan et al., *Surface Modification of Co–Cr Alloy for Orthopaedic Applications*,
Biomedical Materials for Multi-functional Applications,
https://doi.org/10.1007/978-981-95-4029-7_1

bones, cells, and their molecular components, especially in clinical settings where patient outcomes are paramount.

Biomaterials have been widely adopted in various surgical interventions, spanning orthopedics, plastic and reconstructive surgery, dental implants, neurosurgery, cardiovascular procedures, and even veterinary applications. This widespread use underscores the importance of a thorough understanding of the interdisciplinary nature of biomaterials research. Moreover, achieving precise dimensional accuracy and optimizing surface properties of implants are vital factors in ensuring successful integration between the implant and bodily tissues during surgical procedures. The interplay of these elements plays a fundamental role in enhancing the effectiveness and longevity of medical treatments, ultimately contributing to improved patient outcomes and quality of life. As research in this field continues to advance, the potential for innovative biomaterials to further revolutionize medicine appears boundless.

1.2 Properties of Biomaterials

The effectiveness of a biomaterial or implant is influenced by several critical factors, including its structural integrity, chemical composition, mechanical strength, and its interactions with biological systems. Implants, by design, are in direct contact with human tissues, which makes both their mechanical performance and biocompatibility vital for success. Mechanical performance refers to the implant's ability to withstand forces without deforming or failing, while biocompatibility encompasses how well the material integrates with biological tissues without causing adverse reactions. To ensure optimal functionality, it is essential to achieve a delicate balance between the bulk characteristics, such as density and porosity, and the surface properties, including roughness and chemical reactivity, of biomaterials. This balance is crucial for promoting good tissue integration, enhancing cellular responses, and reducing the risk of inflammation or rejection by the body. Various key attributes must be rigorously evaluated when selecting appropriate biomaterials for specific applications [6]. These attributes include the material's mechanical properties, degradation rates, and the ability to support cell attachment and growth. Figure 1.1 illustrates these important factors, providing a visual representation of the considerations necessary for the successful design and application of biomaterials in medical implants.

1.2.1 Physical Properties

In recent years, researchers have increasingly focused on physics-based approaches to enhance the biological responses elicited by biomaterials. The physical characteristics of these materials, such as surface texture, shape, and size, play a significant role in determining how cells interact with them, influencing crucial cellular activities

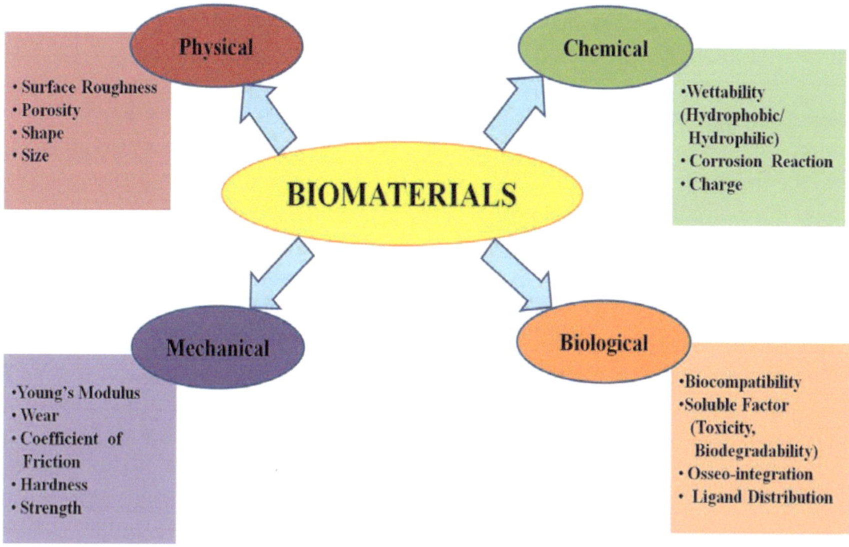

Fig. 1.1 Essential properties of biomaterials

such as adhesion, phagocytosis, proliferation, and targeted interactions. When cells come into contact with a biomaterial's surface, a variety of complex physicochemical interactions occur. These interactions are not solely dependent on the biomaterial itself but are also influenced by a range of factors, including environmental conditions (such as pH and temperature) and cellular behaviors (such as viability and proliferation rates). Among the numerous characteristics of biomaterials, physical and surface parameters, such as morphology, dimensional scale, porosity, and surface texture, are key to determining how effectively a biomaterial functions within biological systems [7].

In particular, particle size is a critical parameter that defines the physical profile of biomaterials. This parameter is crucial in applications like targeted drug delivery and medical imaging, where even slight variations in particle size and distribution can significantly affect the efficacy of the treatment or imaging technique. For instance, nanoparticles may facilitate enhanced drug absorption and cellular uptake, while larger particles may be more suitable for specific imaging applications. In biomedical applications, a range of particle sizes, from the nanometer scale, which allows for deep tissue penetration, to several tens of micrometers, which may enhance delivery to specific sites, has been shown to yield optimal performance [8, 9]. Understanding how these variations impact biological interactions is essential for advancing the development of effective biomaterials for clinical use. As such, ongoing research aims to uncover the intricate relationships between the physical properties of biomaterials and their biological effects, paving the way for innovative applications in medicine and therapeutics [10, 11].

Another important characteristic of biomaterials is the shape of the particles, which significantly affects cell interactions and determines the material's suitability for various biomedical applications [12]. Research has shown that using non-spherical geometries, such as elliptical, cylindrical, or even more complex forms, can provide distinct advantages, particularly in drug delivery systems. These shapes enhance the material's ability to navigate through biological systems, improve drug retention, and optimize release profiles [13, 14]. Moreover, the porosity of biomaterials is a critical factor that influences several cellular processes, including proliferation, adhesion, and migration. Porous structures can mimic the natural extracellular matrix, thereby providing mechanical support, fostering tissue development, and enhancing the integration between the implant and surrounding biological tissues. The interconnected pores allow for the diffusion of nutrients and waste products, which is essential for cell survival and function. Surface roughness also plays a crucial role in determining the effectiveness of biomedical implants. The texture of a surface can substantially impact cell attachment and behavior, affecting how tissues respond to the implant. While smooth surfaces may facilitate easier initial cell adhesion, rough surfaces are generally favored for their ability to promote superior cellular proliferation and tissue integration. The roughness is usually quantified using profilometry techniques, providing precise measurements that can inform design choices. In addition to particle shape, porosity, and surface roughness, other structural factors, such as compartmentalization and material density, also influence the functional performance of biomaterials in biological environments [15]. For instance, compartmentalized structures may allow for the controlled release of therapeutic agents, while variations in material density can affect mechanical properties and biocompatibility, ultimately impacting the longevity and success of the implant within the body. By considering these multiple factors, researchers can better design biomaterials tailored for specific medical applications, ensuring improved patient outcomes.

1.2.2 Chemical Properties

The chemical properties of biomaterials play a crucial role in determining their reactivity and long-term stability, which are essential factors for their effectiveness in medical applications. At the atomic level, the specific arrangement and bonding of atoms within the material profoundly influence its chemical behavior, particularly for biomedical implants that must interact safely and effectively with the human body [16]. These chemical characteristics directly impact a range of biological responses, including cell adhesion, which is the initial attachment of cells to the implant surface; cellular growth, which involves the proliferation and differentiation of cells; and protein adsorption, the process by which proteins adhere to the implant. These interactions are critical for the implant's integration into the body and its ultimate function. Several key chemical attributes define biomaterials, including their susceptibility to corrosion, surface wettability, and the nature of their electrical surface charge. Corrosion is a particularly significant concern for implants intended for long-term placement within the body, as it can compromise their structural integrity and biocompatibility [17, 18]. The biological environment surrounding the implant is complex, comprising components such as blood, interstitial fluids, amino acids, proteins, sodium, and chloride ions. This environment can initiate various electrochemical reactions on the implant's surface, a process known as biocorrosion or fretting corrosion. These reactions can lead to the degradation of the material and negatively affect the implant's longevity [19]. Different forms of corrosion can manifest in biomedical applications, including uniform corrosion, intergranular corrosion, galvanic corrosion which arises when two dissimilar metals come into electrical contact in the presence of an electrolyte, stress corrosion cracking which caused by the combination of tensile stress and a corrosive environment and leads to the crack formation, pitting corrosion, and fatigue corrosion. Understanding these corrosion mechanisms is vital for the development of safer and more durable biomaterials, ultimately improving the outcomes of medical implants and devices [20].

Surface wettability is a critical chemical parameter that significantly impacts biological interactions and the overall performance of biomaterials. Wettability describes how a liquid interacts with a solid surface, specifically how it spreads or adheres, which is primarily influenced by the intermolecular forces between the solid and liquid phases [21]. This interaction is essential in various applications, including medical implants, coatings, and biosensors. Surfaces are classified into two main categories based on their wettability: hydrophilic (water-attracting) and hydrophobic (water-repelling). Hydrophilic surfaces tend to have low contact angles, allowing water to spread easily across the surface, while hydrophobic surfaces have high contact angles, causing water droplets to bead up and minimize contact. The contact angle is a critical measurement that helps to categorize a surface's wettability and can be pivotal in predicting how a biomaterial will interact with bodily fluids and cells. One important aspect of wettability is its effect on protein adsorption, a crucial step in determining biocompatibility. Research has shown that hydrophobic surfaces generally promote greater protein adsorption compared to hydrophilic surfaces. This increased adsorption occurs because hydrophobic interactions facilitate the adherence of hydrophobic regions of proteins to the surface, which can enhance cell attachment and proliferation. In addition to wettability, the surface charge of a biomaterial significantly influences its biocompatibility and cellular responses. The surface charge can attract or repel charged biomolecules, affecting how cells interact with the material. Studies indicate that surfaces with a positive electrical charge often enhance cell attachment and growth compared to neutral or negatively charged surfaces [22]. This positive charge can promote the adsorption of serum proteins that are essential for cell adhesion, ultimately leading to better integration of the biomaterial with surrounding tissues. Understanding the interplay between wettability, surface charge, and protein adsorption is essential for the design of biomaterials that can effectively promote desired biological responses and improve clinical outcomes.

1.2.3 Mechanical Properties

It is essential that the mechanical properties of biomaterials closely align with those of the target tissue or organ, as this compatibility plays a vital role in facilitating cellular adaptation and integration. To achieve effective integration, key mechanical parameters such as Young's modulus, ultimate tensile strength, and toughness must be meticulously evaluated during the selection process of biomaterials. This is particularly important because various human tissues exhibit unique mechanical behaviors and characteristics. For example, soft tissues, such as brain tissue, typically display an elasticity range between approximately 0.1–1 kPa, which allows for the flexibility and compliance necessary to accommodate dynamic physiological functions. In contrast, mineralized bone exhibits significantly higher elasticity, generally starting at around 30 kPa and extending much higher, which contributes to its ability to bear mechanical loads effectively [23]. A critical consideration in the selection of implant materials is the phenomenon known as stress shielding. This occurs when an implant diverts the normal mechanical load away from the surrounding bone. As a result, the bone experiences reduced mechanical stimulation, leading to a decrease in bone density and potential complications such as bone resorption [24]. Studies led by Ibrahim et al. [25] have shown that bones tend to lose mass and structural integrity when they are not subjected to regular loading, which underscores the importance of mechanical compatibility. To mitigate the risk of bone degeneration, it is advisable to select implant materials with a Young's modulus that closely matches that of the native bone. This alignment helps to ensure an even distribution of mechanical stresses across the bone and the implant interface, thereby maintaining the structural integrity of the bone and supporting overall bone health. Additionally, implants should possess high strength values, including both yield strength and compressive strength, in order to withstand the mechanical forces experienced during everyday activities and to ensure mechanical durability over the long term. A thorough comparison of the mechanical properties of various metallic biomaterials against those of natural bone is provided in Table 1.1, offering valuable insights for selecting appropriate materials for specific applications in biomedical engineering [26].

Table 1.1 Mechanical properties of metallic implant materials and natural bone

Mechanical properties	Stainless steel	Ti alloy	Mg alloy	Co–Cr alloy	Natural bone
Modulus elasticity (GPa)	190	110	44	210	3–20
Yield strength (MPa)	331	485	162	448–648	77–114
Tensile strength (MPa)	586	760	250	951–1220	42–109
Fracture toughness ($MPa\sqrt{m}$)	~ 100	~ 80	15–40	~ 100	2–12
Density (g/cm^3)	7.9	4.5	1.84	9.2	1.8–2.1

Reproduced with permission from Elsevier [26]

Wear resistance is a crucial mechanical property that describes the gradual deterioration of material from a surface as a result of mechanical interactions with another surface. This attribute is particularly important in biomedical applications, as the wear and friction behavior of biomaterials can significantly impact both their functional lifespan and overall mechanical reliability [27]. When wear occurs, it can lead to the release of metallic particles or ions at the interface between the bone and the implant. Such releases are not merely a mechanical concern; they can provoke negative biological responses, potentially compromising the success of the implant and the health of surrounding tissues. To thoroughly assess the wear characteristics of biomaterials, researchers employ various experimental techniques [28]. Notable among these are the ball-on-disk, pin-on-disk, and block-on-disk methods. Each of these techniques simulates different contact conditions and loading scenarios that materials might encounter in real-world applications, allowing for a comprehensive evaluation of wear resistance. By understanding these wear mechanisms and employing rigorous testing methods, engineers can design biomaterials that are not only durable but also biocompatible, thereby enhancing the longevity and safety of implants in clinical use.

When selecting materials for implants, it is essential that they possess low friction properties and high resistance to wear. These characteristics are crucial for ensuring the longevity and effectiveness of the implants within the body. Key mechanical properties, particularly hardness and toughness, must be thoroughly assessed as they significantly impact the performance of biomaterials. Hardness refers to a material's ability to withstand deformation and abrasion, making it a vital property for minimizing wear. Implants with increased hardness are less prone to surface degradation, which can ultimately lead to implant failure. On the other hand, toughness, or tenacity, is the material's ability to absorb energy and deform without fracturing. Enhanced toughness is important because it provides greater resistance to fractures, which can occur under the stresses experienced in biological environments. In summary, a careful evaluation of these mechanical properties, hardness to prevent wear and toughness to prevent fractures, is critical in the development and selection of effective biomaterials for medical implants. This ensures not only the durability of the implants but also the safety and well-being of patients.

1.2.4 Biological Properties

The development of biomaterials is intricately linked to their biological performance, particularly when they are implanted in the human body. Upon implantation, these materials are exposed to a complex biological environment that includes various cell types, proteins, and biological fluids. Therefore, it becomes crucial to carefully consider several key attributes during the design phase to ensure the biomaterial's long-term effectiveness and success. One of the primary attributes is biocompatibility, which refers to a material's ability to interact safely with human tissues and organs without eliciting harmful effects or adverse immune reactions [29]. A biocompatible material must be non-toxic and should not release particles or chemical substances that may provoke immune responses, inflammation, or other negative physiological reactions in tissues or biological fluids. This property is essential for minimizing the risk of complications post-implantation. Other critical factors include osseointegration, which is the process by which the biomaterial integrates with the surrounding bone tissue, allowing for stable support and functionality. Biodegradability is also important, as it refers to the material's ability to break down safely over time within the body, often transforming into non-toxic byproducts that can be easily metabolized or excreted. Additionally, ligand distribution plays a significant role in how well a biomaterial interacts at the molecular level with surrounding biological tissues. This aspect can influence cell adhesion, proliferation, and differentiation, thus affecting the overall success of the implant. To evaluate the compatibility of biomaterials with living organisms, researchers typically conduct in-vitro (testing in controlled environments outside of a living organism) or in-vivo (testing within a living organism) assessments. These rigorous testing protocols provide valuable insights into the material's performance and its potential interactions with biological systems, ensuring that they meet the necessary standards for clinical applications.

A variety of standardized methods are employed to thoroughly evaluate the biological behavior of materials, particularly in the context of medical implants and prosthetic devices. These evaluation techniques encompass cytotoxicity assays, hemocompatibility assessments, implantation studies, and tests for irritation and sensitization. Cytotoxicity testing is a crucial step in determining how materials affect living cells. It often involves measuring cell viability through several approaches, including direct contact with the material, indirect exposure through culture medium, or using assays such as the MTT assay, which assesses metabolic activity as an indicator of cell health. This testing helps identify any potential toxic effects that materials may have on surrounding tissues. Hemocompatibility assessments focus on how well materials interact with blood, which is vital for implants that will be placed in vascular environments. These assessments evaluate parameters such as blood coagulation, platelet activation, and any adverse reactions that might occur upon contact with blood, ensuring that the material will not provoke an inflammatory response. Implantation studies provide insights into the long-term performance of materials once they are inserted into the body. Researchers observe how the body reacts to the implant over time, monitoring for signs of rejection, integration, and overall functionality [30]. Sensitization tests are designed to detect any potential allergic reactions that could occur when the material interacts with the body's immune system. These tests ensure that materials are safe for clinical use and do not elicit undesirable immune responses. Osseointegration, a key concept in implantology, refers to the process of achieving a stable and direct connection between the surface of an implant and the surrounding bone tissue, with no intervening soft tissue layer. This process is critical for the success of load-bearing implants, such as those used in dental or orthopedic applications [31]. Several key factors significantly influence the success of osseointegration. These include the surface chemistry of the implant, its roughness, and the topographical features of its surface. Materials that promote effective bonding between the implant and bone tissue not only enhance mechanical stability but also improve the functional longevity of bioinert materials. This, in turn, leads to better performance outcomes for prosthetic devices, significantly impacting patient satisfaction and quality of life [32, 33]. In summary, a comprehensive understanding of these assessment methods and factors affecting osseointegration is essential for the successful development and implementation of biocompatible materials in medical applications.

Biodegradability is a fundamental characteristic of materials, specifically referring to their ability to break down, dissolve, or be absorbed by biological systems over time. This property is particularly advantageous in the context of medical implants, as it reduces the necessity for additional surgical procedures to remove these devices once the healing process is complete. By designing implants that naturally degrade within the body, healthcare providers can minimize patient discomfort and the risks associated with subsequent surgeries. Furthermore, the spatial distribution of ligands, whether they are found within cells (intracellular) or outside of them (extracellular), significantly influences how biomaterials interact with biological systems. This spatial arrangement can modulate various biological responses, including cell adhesion, proliferation, and differentiation, ultimately affecting the success of the implant. In addition to biodegradability and ligand distribution, several other vital properties must be optimized to enhance the performance of biomaterials used in medical applications. These include biocompatibility, which ensures that the material does not provoke an adverse immune response; bio-inertness, which allows for a passive interaction with surrounding tissues; and bioactivity, which facilitates beneficial biological responses. By carefully balancing these traits, researchers can improve the lifespan and overall efficiency of biomaterials, ensuring they function effectively as implants within the human body [34].

1.3 Types of Biomaterials

Biomaterials, which are essential in the field of medicine, can be categorized based on their structural, chemical, and biological properties into several specific classes. These include ceramics, glasses, metals, polymers, and composite materials. Each class exhibits unique attributes and varying levels of bioactivity, which play a crucial role in determining their suitability for various medical applications. This classification is illustrated in Table 1.2, which provides a diverse biomaterials and their biological responses. Among these materials, metallic implants have emerged as vital components in the repair and regeneration of both long bones and soft tissues within the human body. Their robust mechanical properties, resistance to deformation, and ability to support physiological loads make metals, like titanium and stainless steel, particularly valuable in orthopedic surgery. However, the history of metallic implants is fraught with challenges.

In the 1860s, early attempts to employ metallic substances such as iron, gold, or silver for spinal wires and bone pins yielded disappointing results. These materials

Table 1.2 Types of biomaterials and their applications

Synthetic biomaterials	Applications
Metals	Orthopedic devices, dental implants
Polymers	Ocular implants, drug delivery devices skin/cartilage
Ceramics	Bones replacements, heart valves, dental implants
Semi-conductors	Biosensor, implantable microelectrodes

were often rejected by the body's immune system, leading to significant complications, including severe post-surgical infections that hindered recovery and resulted in poor patient outcomes. Amidst these challenges, Scottish surgeon Joseph Lister introduced a revolutionary approach to surgical practice that transformed the landscape of medicine. Lister's pioneering work in aseptic surgery emphasized the importance of maintaining a sterile environment during surgical procedures. By utilizing carbolic acid as an antiseptic, he significantly reduced the incidence of infections that plagued surgical patients. His methods not only changed the standard of care but also laid the groundwork for modern surgical techniques [6]. Lister's emphasis on cleanliness and aseptic techniques became a foundational principle in surgery, ultimately leading to improved surgical outcomes and the establishment of protocols that prioritize patient safety. His legacy continues to influence surgical practices today, highlighting the critical intersection of biomaterial development and surgical innovation.

Over the years, metallic materials have become fundamental in orthopedic and dental applications, playing a critical role in improving patient outcomes. These materials are utilized in a wide array of devices, which include temporary fixation tools such as bone plates, screws, and hooks that aid in stabilizing fractures and ensuring proper healing. Additionally, they are instrumental in permanent implants like total joint replacements, which help restore mobility and functionality to patients suffering from degenerative joint diseases or injuries [35, 36]. Among the metals commonly used in these biomedical applications are stainless steel, titanium, magnesium, and cobalt-chromium alloys, each chosen for its unique properties that meet the specific demands of medical use [37]. Notably, 316L stainless steel has emerged as a particularly popular choice since its introduction in the 1920s. This alloy is favored for its exceptional mechanical properties, corrosion resistance, and compatibility with the human body, making it suitable for a wide range of medical devices and implants. Recent studies have highlighted the significant role of 316L stainless steel in hip replacement surgeries, with approximately 70% of Orthinox stainless steel being utilized for these procedures in the United States. This statistic underscores the alloy's importance in orthopedic surgery [38]. 316L stainless steel primarily consists of iron and comprises between 11 and 30% chromium by weight, along with varying amounts of nickel, all of which contribute to its strength, durability, and resistance to corrosion in the bodily environment [39]. As research and technology advance, the development of metallic materials continues to evolve, promising even greater innovations in patient care and surgical outcomes.

Stainless steel is typically categorized into four primary types based on their unique crystal structures: martensitic (body-centered tetragonal, known for its hardness), ferritic (body-centered cubic), austenitic (face-centered cubic), and duplex (a combination of austenitic and ferritic phases), as outlined in Table 1.3 [35]. Duplex stainless steels offer high strength and enhanced resistance to stress corrosion cracking, making them advantageous for demanding environments. The significance of martensitic, ferritic, and austenitic stainless steels in the biomedical sector can be attributed to their combination of essential features. These materials are valued for their widespread availability, cost-effectiveness, and ease of fabrication, which streamline the manufacturing process of medical devices. Moreover, their reliable biocompatibility ensures safety when interacting with biological tissues, while their mechanical toughness allows them to withstand the physical stresses encountered in various medical applications. Additionally, their high resistance to corrosion ensures longevity and durability in the body, making stainless steel an ideal choice for a range of implantable devices, surgical instruments, and other medical tools [39].

Magnesium was first isolated by Sir Humphry Davy in 1808, marking a significant milestone in material science and paving the way for its subsequent exploration as a biodegradable material in biomedical applications. By the late nineteenth century, advancements in medical technology led to the implementation of magnesium wires and implants in clinical settings. These were utilized for various procedures, particularly in the cardiovascular system, musculoskeletal repairs, fluid drainage, and general surgeries, showcasing magnesium's versatility and potential in the medical field [40]. One of magnesium's key advantages lies in its mechanical properties, specifically its density and elastic modulus, which closely match those of human bone. This similarity not only enhances biocompatibility but also helps reduce the stress-shielding effect, a phenomenon where rigid implant materials, such as stainless steel, cobalt-based alloys, and titanium alloys, can lead to bone resorption and

Table 1.3 Classifications of stainless steels and typical medical applications

Material type (SS)	Application grade	Examples
Martensitic	Dental and surgical instruments	Bone curettes, chisels and gouges, dental burs, dental chisels, curettes, explorers, root elevators and scalers, forceps, hemostats, retractors, orthodontic pliers, and scalpels
Ferritic	Minimal surgical instruments	Solid handles for instruments, guide pins, and fasteners
Austenitic	A large number of non-implantable medical devices. Many short-term implants total hip replacements	Cannula, dental impression trays, guide pins, hollowware, hypodermic needles, steam sterilizers, storage cabinets and work surfaces, and thoracic retractors
Duplex	Not yet applied in the biomedical field	

Reproduced with permission from Taylor & Francis [35]

delayed healing by taking on most of the mechanical load. By using magnesium implants, the load is more evenly distributed, promoting proper bone integration and healing. Furthermore, magnesium's biodegradable nature means that it can gradually dissolve in the body, eliminating the need for a second surgical procedure to remove the implant, which is an additional consideration in patient care and recovery. This combination of properties positions magnesium as a promising alternative in the development of future biomedical implants [41, 42].

One major advantage of magnesium is its unique ability to degrade naturally within the body (in-vivo). This characteristic eliminates the necessity for a secondary surgical procedure to remove the implant, as the degradation byproducts are efficiently expelled through urine. This natural process not only simplifies post-operative care but also reduces the associated risks and discomfort of additional surgeries [43]. Moreover, magnesium ions (Mg^{2+}) play a crucial role in promoting the formation of new trabecular bone and have been demonstrated to accelerate the healing process of fractures. This regenerative capability makes magnesium a valuable material in orthopedic applications, particularly for patients recovering from bone injuries or surgeries [44]. Research indicates that the human body typically absorbs between 250 and 500 mg of magnesium daily, primarily through dietary sources and normal physiological functions. In an average adult weighing around 70 kg, the total body content of magnesium is estimated to be approximately 20 g. While the body requires magnesium for various essential functions, including muscle contraction, nerve transmission, and energy production, a definitive toxic threshold has yet to be established, underscoring the need for further research in this area [45]. In addition to its biological benefits, magnesium possesses several advantageous physical properties that enhance its utility in various applications. These include: (a) a high strength-to-weight ratio, which makes it an ideal choice for lightweight structural components; (b) excellent thermal and electrical conductivity, facilitating its use in electronic devices and heat sinks; (c) effective vibration damping and shock absorption, making it suitable for use in automotive and aerospace applications; (d) high damping capacity, which reduces noise and enhances comfort in products; and (e) efficient electromagnetic shielding, which protects sensitive electronics from interference [46–48]. These properties collectively position magnesium as a versatile and valuable material in both medical and industrial fields, highlighting its potential for innovative applications in future.

Titanium began to gain significant recognition in the late 1940s for its promising potential in surgical applications. Researchers quickly turned their attention to evaluating its biocompatibility and suitability as material for implants [49, 50]. Initially, the use of titanium was primarily limited to a few countries, including the United States and the United Kingdom, where the medical community began to explore its unique properties. What sets titanium apart are its exceptional characteristics: it has a low elastic modulus, which allows it to mimic the mechanical properties of bone, thereby reducing the likelihood of implant failure. Additionally, titanium displays excellent corrosion resistance, crucial for medical implants that must remain stable within the human body for long periods. Its high biocompatibility means that titanium is less likely to provoke an immune response, making it an ideal choice for various biomedical applications. Over the years, titanium has become widely accepted in numerous medical fields, particularly in dental implants, orthopedic devices, and electronic implants, where reliability and longevity are critical [51, 52]. Its high specific strength, defined as the strength-to-density ratio, enables titanium to form stable, long-lasting bonds with surrounding bone tissue. This superior bonding ability allows titanium to outperform traditional materials like stainless steel and cobalt alloys in numerous applications, including hip, knee, shoulder, spine, and wrist implants [53]. A notable recent advancement in the field involved the Australian medical device company CSIRO, which successfully implanted a 3D-printed titanium sternum and rib cage into a patient suffering from chest wall sarcoma (Fig. 1.2d) [54]. This groundbreaking procedure demonstrates not only the versatility of titanium as a material but also the potential of advanced manufacturing techniques in revolutionizing personalized medicine and improving patient outcomes.

Cobalt-chromium (Co–Cr) alloys are extensively utilized as metallic biomaterials, particularly for permanent joint replacements in both orthopedic and dental applications. Their journey began with dental implants but broadened significantly in the 1940s when they were adopted for use in artificial hips and knees. The primary

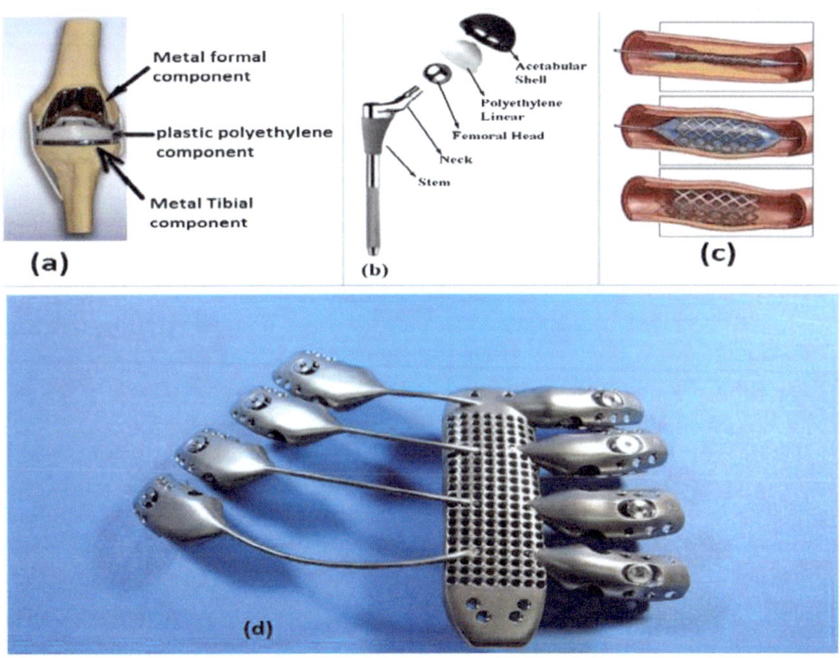

Fig. 1.2 Some applications of biomaterial in different biological systems **a** artificial knee joint comprises metallic (Ti or Co–Cr alloys) and UHMW polymer component; **b** hip joint comprises metallic, polymers and high wear resistant ceramic component; **c** mesh type stent for coronary artery and **d** 3D printed sternum and rib cage of titanium alloy. Reproduced with permission from Taylor & Francis [35]

components of these alloys are cobalt, chromium, and molybdenum, each playing a crucial role in their performance and durability [55]. Chromium and cobalt work together to enhance the corrosion resistance of Co–Cr alloys. They achieve this by forming a passive oxide layer on the surface, which protects the underlying material from degradation in the corrosive environment of the human body. This passive layer is vital for the long-term success of implants, as it helps prevent wear and potential release of metal ions into the surrounding tissue. Molybdenum further complements these properties by improving the mechanical strength of the alloys and refining the grain structure, resulting in a material that can withstand the mechanical stresses encountered in joint applications [56]. In physiological conditions, cobalt and chromium exist at concentrations typically below 0.25 μg/L in the human body, indicating that these metals are generally safe when used in biocompatible applications. Over the last fifty years, Co–Cr alloys have established themselves as highly reliable biomaterials, backed by extensive clinical experience. Variants such as F75 (Co–Cr–Mo), F90 (Co–Cr–W–Ni), and F562 (Co–Ni–Cr–Mo) are commonly employed in various medical fields. These specific formulations are chosen for their robust mechanical properties, excellent biocompatibility, and superior resistance to wear and corrosion. The versatility of Co–Cr alloys allows them to excel in demanding environments, such as those found in joint replacements and dental appliances, where the combination of strength, durability, and safety is paramount [57, 58]. As research continues to evolve, the applications of Co–Cr alloys are likely to expand even further, reinforcing their position as a cornerstone of modern biomedical engineering.

Polymeric biomaterials, commonly referred to as biopolymers, have gained significant traction in the biomedical field due to their remarkable versatility and adaptability across various applications. These materials are essential in creating contact lenses that ensure comfort and oxygen permeability, drug delivery systems designed to optimize therapeutic effects, and advanced techniques for tissue and muscle repair. Additionally, biopolymers are integral in developing bone fixation devices, such as screws, that provide stable support for healing fractures. The two primary categories of biopolymers include naturally derived polymers, such as silk, which is prized for its strength and biocompatibility; cellulose, known for its biodegradability and abundance; and chitosan, recognized for its antimicrobial properties; and synthetic polymers like nylon and polystyrene, which are engineered to meet specific medical requirements [59]. These materials play central roles in tissue engineering and regenerative medicine, facilitating the growth and repair of tissues by acting as scaffolds that promote cell attachment and proliferation. Beyond polymers, ceramic and glass-based materials are extensively utilized in biomedical applications, primarily due to their exceptional chemical stability, mechanical strength, and compatibility with biological tissues [60]. Bioceramics, in particular, are vital for enhancing the performance of metallic implants, such as hip and knee prostheses. They provide protective coatings that not only improve wear resistance but also reduce the risk of inflammation and rejection by the body's immune system. Common applications of bioceramics encompass a wide range of medical needs, including dental prosthetics, where they offer durable and aesthetically pleasing solutions; bone grafts that assist in the reconstruction of damaged bones; artificial heart valves that ensure proper blood flow; and surgical bone cements that bond prosthetics to the existing bone structure effectively [61]. By integrating these advanced materials, the field of biomedical engineering continues to evolve, improving patient outcomes and advancing our understanding of tissue regeneration and repair.

Semiconductor-based technologies are gaining significant attention in the field of tissue engineering due to their innovative capabilities. These technologies can be seamlessly embedded within various biomaterials, enabling them to capture physiological signals in the form of electrical outputs. This integration facilitates real-time monitoring and assessment of implant functionality and performance, which is crucial for improving patient outcomes and the longevity of implants. By harnessing the sensitivity and precision of semiconductor components, researchers can enhance the design of implants, allowing for more effective responses to the body's physiological changes. This real-time feedback system not only improves the understanding of how implants interact with biological tissues but also aids in optimizing their performance over time [62]. Representative examples of commonly used implantable biomaterials that incorporate these advanced technologies are illustrated in Fig. 1.2. These materials highlight the potential for synergistic applications that can lead to more successful tissue engineering outcomes.

References

1. Ferrer-Miralles N, Rodriguez-Carmona E, Corchero JL, Garcia-Fruitos E, Vazquez E, Villaverde A (2015) Engineering protein self-assembling in protein-based nanomedicines for drug delivery and gene therapy. Crit Rev Biotechnol 35(2):209–221
2. Boretos JW, Eden M (1984) Contemporary biomaterials: material and host response, clinical applications, new technology and legal aspects. J Membr Sci 21:209
3. Patel NR, Gohil PP (2012) A review on biomaterials: scope, applications & human anatomy significance. Int J Emerg Technol Adv Eng 2(4):91–101
4. Langer R, Tirrell DA (2004) Designing materials for biology and medicine. Nature 428(6982):487–492
5. Shi D (2006) Introduction to biomaterials, 1st edn. World Scientific Publishing Co, Beijing, p 3
6. Park J, Lakes RS (2007) Biomaterials: an introduction, 3rd edn. Springer Science and Business Media, Berlin, p 5
7. Mitragotri S, Lahann J (2009) Physical approaches to biomaterial design. Nat Mater 8(1):15
8. Gao H, Shi W, Freund LB (2005) Mechanics of receptor-mediated endocytosis. Proc Natl Acad Sci USA 102:9469–9474
9. Singh M, Chakrapani A, O'Hagan D (2007) Nanoparticles and microparticles as vaccine-delivery systems. Expert Rev Vaccines 6:797–808
10. Alexis F, Pridgen E, Molnar LK, Farokhzad OC (2008) Factors affecting the clearance and biodistribution of polymeric nanoparticles. Mol Pharmacol 5:505–515
11. Kohane DS (2007) Microparticles and nanoparticles for drug delivery. Biotechnol Bioeng 96:203–209
12. Champion JA, Katare YK, Mitragotri S (2007) Particle shape: a new design parameter for micro- and nanoscale drug delivery carriers. J Control Release 121:3–9
13. Decuzzi P, Ferrari M (2006) The adhesive strength of non-spherical particles mediated by specific interactions. Biomaterials 27:5307–5314

14. Decuzzi P, Ferrari M (2008) The receptor-mediated endocytosis of non-spherical particles. Biophys J 94:3790–3797
15. Wieland M, Chehroudi B, Textor M, Brunette DM (2002) Use of Ti-coated replicas to investigate the effects on fibroblast shape of surfaces with varying roughness and constant chemical composition. J Biomed Mater Res 60(3):434–444
16. Santos VD, Brandalise RN, Savaris M (2017) Biomaterials: characteristics and properties. In: Engineering of biomaterials. Springer, Cham, pp 5–15
17. Fraker AC (1987) ASM handbook, 9th edn. ASM International, pp 1324–1335
18. Kubie LS, Shult GM (1925) Studies on the relationship of the chemical constituents of blood and cerebrospinal fluid. J Exp Med 42:565–591
19. Singh R, Dahotre NB (2007) Corrosion degradation and prevention by surface modification of biometallic materials. J Mater Sci 18:725–751
20. Gilbert JL (2017) Corrosion in the human body: metallic implants in the complex body environment. Corrosion 73(12):1478–1495
21. Xu LC, Siedlecki CA (2007) Effects of surface wettability and contact time on protein adhesion to biomaterial surfaces. Biomaterials 28(22):3273–3283
22. Chang HI, Wang Y (2011) Cell responses to surface and architecture of tissue engineering scaffolds. In: Eberli D (ed) Regenerative medicine and tissue engineering—cells and biomaterials, pp 569–588
23. Rehfeldt F, Engler AJ, Eckhardt A, Ahmed F, Discher DE (2007) Cell responses to the mechanochemical microenvironment: implications for regenerative medicine and drug delivery. Adv Drug Deliv Rev 59:1329–1339
24. Ridzwan MIZ, Shuib S, Hassan AY, Shokri AA, Ibrahim MM (2007) Problem of stress shielding and improvement to the hip implant designs: a review. J Med Sci 7(3):460–467
25. Ibrahim H, Esfahani SN, Poorganji B, Dean D, Elahinia M (2017) Resorbable bone fixation alloys, forming, and post-fabrication treatments. Mater Sci Eng C 70:870–888
26. Yang J, Cui FZ, Lee IS, Wang X (2010) Plasma surface modification of magnesium alloy for biomedical application. Surf Coat Technol 205:S182–S187
27. Alvarado J, Maldonado R, Marxuach J, Otero R (2003) Biomechanics of hip and knee prostheses. In: Applications of engineering mechanics in medicine. GED-University of Puerto Rico, Mayaguez, pp 1–20
28. Roychowdhury A, Gupta S, Vidyasagara PEC, Pal S (2004) Wear studies of frequently used implant materials. Trends Biomater Artif Organs 17:135–140
29. Williams DF (1986) Definitions in biomaterials: proceedings of a consensus conference of the European society for biomaterials, vol 4. Elsevier Science Limited, Chester
30. Qin Y (2015) Biocompatibility testing for medical textile products. Medical textile materials, 1st edn. Woodhead Publishing, Cambridge, pp 191–201
31. Nasab MB, Hassan MR (2010) Metallic biomaterials of knee and hip—a review. Trends Biomater Artif Organs 24:69–82
32. Parsapour A, Khorasani SN, Fathi MH (2012) Effect of surface treatment and metallic coating on corrosion behavior and biocompatibility of surgical 316L stainless steel implant. J Mater Sci Technol 28(2):125–131
33. Subramanian B, Ananthakumar R, Kobayashi A, Jayachandran M (2012) Surface modification of 316L stainless steel with magnetron sputtered TiN/VN nanoscale multilayers for bio implant applications. J Mater Sci Mater Med 23(2):329–338
34. Hench LL, Wilson J (1999) An introduction to bioceramics. World Scientific Publish, Singapore
35. Chen Q, Thouas GA (2015) Metallic implant biomaterials. Mater Sci Eng R 87:1–57
36. Rupp F, Geis-Gerstorfer J, Geckeler KE (1996) Dental implant materials: surface modification and interface phenomena. Adv Mater 8:254–257
37. Bose S, Banerjee D, Bandyopadhyay A (2017) Materials for bone disorders, 1st edn. Academic Press, London, UK, pp 1–27
38. Rokkum M, Bye K, Hetland KR, Reigstad A (1995) Stem fracture with the exeter prosthesis 3 of 27 hips followed for 10 years. Acta Orthop Scand 66:435–439

39. Davis JR (2003) Metallic materials. In: Handbook of materials for medical devices, 1st edn. ASM International, Geauga, pp 22–30
40. Witte F (2010) The history of biodegradable magnesium implants: a review. Acta Biomater 6:1680–1692
41. Staiger MP, Pietak AM, Huadmai J, Dias G (2006) Magnesium and its alloys as orthopedic biomaterials: a review. Biomaterials 27:1728–1734
42. Zeng R, Dietzel W, Witte F, Hort N, Blawert C (2008) Progress and challenge for magnesium alloys as biomaterials. Adv Eng Mater 10:B3–B14
43. Hermawan H, Dube D, Mantovani D (2010) Developments in metallic biodegradable stent. Acta Biomater 6:1693–1697
44. Hornberger H, Virtanen S, Boccaccini AR (2012) Biomedical coatings on magnesium alloys—a review. Acta Biomater 8(7):2442–2455
45. Rude RK (1998) Magnesium deficiency: a cause of heterogeneous disease in humans. J Bone Miner Res 13:749–758
46. Eliezer D, Aghion E, Froes FS (1998) Magnesium science, technology and applications. Adv Perform Mater 5:201–212
47. James DW (1969) High damping metals for engineering applications. Mater Sci Eng 4:1–8
48. Lin BT, Kuo CC (2009) Application of an integrated RE/RP/CAD/CAE/CAM system for magnesium alloy shell of mobile phone. J Mater Process Technol 209:2818–2830
49. Bothe RT, Beaton LE, Davenport HA (1940) Reaction of bone to multiple metallic implants. Surg Gynecol Obstet 71:598–602
50. Niinomi M (1998) Mechanical properties of biomedical titanium alloys. Mater Sci Eng A 243:231–236
51. Wang K (1996) The use of titanium for medical applications in the USA. Mater Sci Eng A 213:134–137
52. Vorobyev AY, Guo C (2007) Femtosecond laser structuring of titanium implants. Appl Surf Sci 253(17):7272–7280
53. Bereznai M, Pelsoczi I, Toth Z, Turzo K, Radnai M, Bor Z, Fazekas A (2003) Surface modifications induced by ns and sub-ps excimer laser pulses on titanium implant material. Biomaterials 24:4197–4203
54. Cancer patient receives 3D printed ribs in world first surgery. Cited 11 Sept 2015. http://www.csiro.au/en/News/News-releases
55. Saini M, Singh Y, Arora P, Arora V, Jain K (2015) Implant biomaterials: a comprehensive review. World J Clin Cases 3:52
56. Manivasagam G, Dhinasekaran D, Rajamanickam A (2010) Biomedical implants: corrosion and its prevention—a review. Recent Pat Corros Sci 2:40–54
57. Mantrala KM, Das M, Balla VK, Rao CS, Rao VK (2014) Laser-deposited CoCrMo alloy: microstructure, wear, and electrochemical properties. J Mater Res 29:2021–2027
58. Tarzia V, Bottio T, Testolin L, Gerosa G (2007) Extended (31 years) durability of Starr–Edwards prosthesis in mitral position. Interact Cardiovasc Thorac Surg 6:570–571
59. Tang X, Thankappan SK, Lee P, Fard SE, Harmon MD, Tran K, Yu X (2014) Polymeric biomaterials in tissue engineering and regenerative medicine. In: Natural and synthetic biomedical polymers, pp 351–371
60. Ducheyne P, Qiu Q (1999) Bioactive ceramics: the effect of surface reactivity on bone formation and bone cell function. Biomaterials 20(23–24):2287–2303
61. Sarkar R, Banerjee G (2010) Ceramic based bio-medical implants. Interceram 59(2):98–102
62. Zimmerman J, Parameswaran R, Tian B (2014) Nanoscale semiconductor devices as new biomaterials. Biomater Sci 2(5):619–626

Chapter 2
Surface Engineering of Metallic Biomaterials

Over the years, extensive research has been dedicated to exploring both metallic and non-metallic biomaterials to develop effective implants for medical use. Despite these efforts, finding a single material that satisfactorily fulfills all biological and mechanical compatibility criteria for integration with the human body remains a complex and unresolved challenge. Implant failures are often attributed to a range of issues. These include inadequate inflammatory responses, which can hinder healing; susceptibility to bacterial infections, which may lead to systemic complications; and mechanical challenges such as corrosion, wear, and loosening of the implant. Such failures not only compromise patient outcomes but also frequently necessitate costly and invasive revision surgeries. To tackle these significant hurdles, surface engineering has emerged as an essential strategy aimed at enhancing the long-term integration and functionality of implants within the biological environment. By modifying the surfaces of biomaterials, researchers can improve biocompatibility, reduce the risk of infection, and promote better bonding with surrounding tissues. This chapter delves into various surface modification techniques employed on commonly used metallic biomaterials, including stainless steel, magnesium, titanium, and cobalt-chromium alloys. We will explore the mechanisms and benefits of these techniques, as well as the implications for the durability and performance of implants in clinical applications. Through this discussion, we aim to shed light on the innovative approaches that are paving the way for the development of more reliable and effective biomedical devices.

2.1 Stainless Steel

Stainless steel is one of the most commonly utilized metals in the manufacturing of medical devices, with significant applications in the orthopedic and dental fields. According to Geanta et al. [1], about 1% of global stainless-steel production is

© The Author(s), under exclusive license to Springer Nature Singapore Pte Ltd. 2026
A. Mahajan et al., *Surface Modification of Co–Cr Alloy for Orthopaedic Applications*, Biomedical Materials for Multi-functional Applications,
https://doi.org/10.1007/978-981-95-4029-7_2

allocated specifically for the creation of surgical instruments and healthcare-related equipment, highlighting the critical role this material plays in modern medicine. Despite its extensive use, stainless steel is not without its challenges. One of the primary concerns is its susceptibility to fissure and fretting corrosion, which can occur when the protective chromium oxide layer, a key feature that imparts corrosion resistance, degrades [2]. This degradation can be exacerbated by factors such as mechanical stress, the presence of bodily fluids, and environmental conditions, ultimately compromising the integrity of the implants. Moreover, without appropriate surface modifications, stainless steel implants can elicit adverse biological responses within the human body [3, 4]. Such reactions can range from inflammation to rejection, making it essential to enhance the biocompatibility of these materials. Advances in surface treatment techniques, such as coating, passivation, and the incorporation of bioactive materials, are being researched and implemented to mitigate these issues and improve the performance and reliability of stainless steel in medical applications.

In a comprehensive study conducted by Hanawa [5], it was observed that stainless steel exhibits a notably slower repassivation rate than other biomaterials. This slower rate signifies a delayed regeneration of the passive oxide layer, which is crucial for protecting the metal from corrosive environments. Figure 2.1 illustrates a detailed comparison of repassivation times required for surface oxide layer formation across various metals and alloys, highlighting the distinct differences in performance between these materials. Further investigations by Sivakumar et al. [6] focused on the common causes of failure in stainless steel implants, as depicted in Fig. 2.2a. Their research identified that fractures are the predominant cause of these implant failures, raising significant concerns regarding the long-term reliability of stainless steel in medical applications. Figure 2.2b provides a distribution of failures across different anatomical regions, revealing that approximately 74% of failures occurred in the femoral region. This concentration of failures suggests that specific anatomical considerations must be taken into account when designing and implementing stainless steel implants. Despite the wealth of research dedicated to surface treatments of materials such as titanium, aluminum, gold, silicon-based substances, and various polymers, the body of work focusing on the surface modification of stainless steel remains comparatively limited [7]. This gap in research underscores the pressing need to explore innovative surface enhancement strategies for stainless steel. Such enhancements could significantly improve the material's performance in critical areas, including chemical stability, mechanical strength, corrosion resistance, biocompatibility, and long-term durability [8]. Addressing these aspects is essential for advancing the use of stainless steel in biomedical applications and enhancing patient outcomes.

Liu et al. [9] developed a water-based sol–gel method for depositing a thin film of hydroxyapatite (HAp) onto the surface of roughened 316L stainless steel. This innovative approach aimed to enhance the biocompatibility of the metal for biomedical applications. While the study identified the presence of microcracks within the HAp coating, which were found to compromise interfacial bonding strength, it was noteworthy that the adhesion performance still surpassed that of traditional plasma-sprayed coatings by approximately 40%. This improvement highlights the

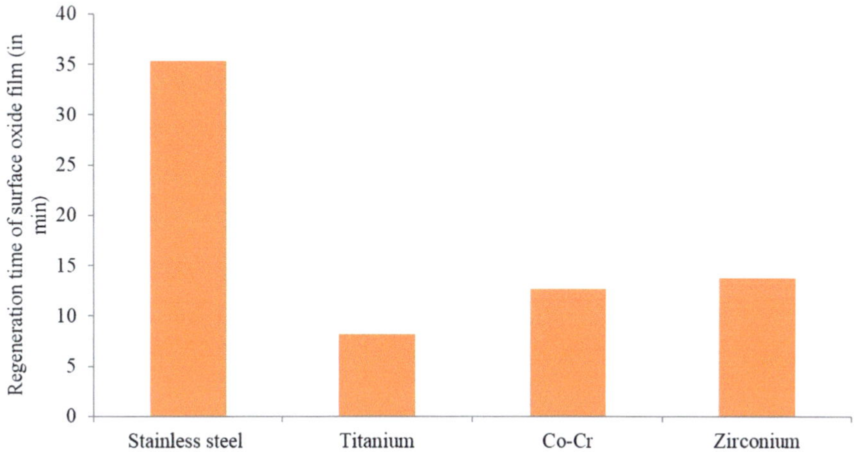

Fig. 2.1 Regeneration time taken by different metals or alloys to develop surface oxide film

potential of sol–gel methods for producing reliable coatings for medical devices. In another investigation, Shih et al. [10] assessed the corrosion behavior of 316L stainless steel wire designed specifically for biomedical use. Their research revealed that a surface treated with an amorphous oxide layer exhibited significantly better corrosion resistance compared to conventional electropolished specimens. This finding suggests that the quality of surface treatment is crucial for enhancing the longevity and functionality of materials used in medical implants.

To address the drawbacks often associated with conventional electropolishing, Abdel-Fattah et al. [11] introduced an electrochemical pretreatment (ECPT) process utilizing a non-acidic ionic liquid medium comprising ethylene glycol and vitamin B4 in a 2:1 ratio. Conducting this treatment at a current density of 0.14 A/cm^2 and a voltage of 1.5 V led to a remarkable 85% reduction in the surface roughness of 316L stainless steel. Such a significant reduction enhances the smoothness of the surface, thereby improving its wear resistance and making it more suitable for biomedical applications. Latifi et al. [12] took a hybrid approach by combining electropolishing with an acid dip process, which yielded an exceptionally smooth, clean, and corrosion-resistant surface. Their method resulted in a greater than 50-fold reduction in surface roughness compared to standard electropolishing alone. This combined technique not only enhanced the aesthetic qualities of the steel but also fortified its resistance to environmental degradation, which is particularly important in the context of medical devices that must endure harsh bodily conditions. Furthering this line of research, Habibzadeh et al. [13] focused on optimizing the electrolyte composition and the applied voltage during the electrochemical polishing of 316L stainless steel. The optimized electrolyte mixture contained 60% phosphoric acid, 20% sulfuric acid, 10% glycerol, and 10% deionized water. Their findings demonstrated that operating at a voltage of 10 V facilitated the formation of a passive oxide film enriched in chromium, significantly enhancing the corrosion resistance,

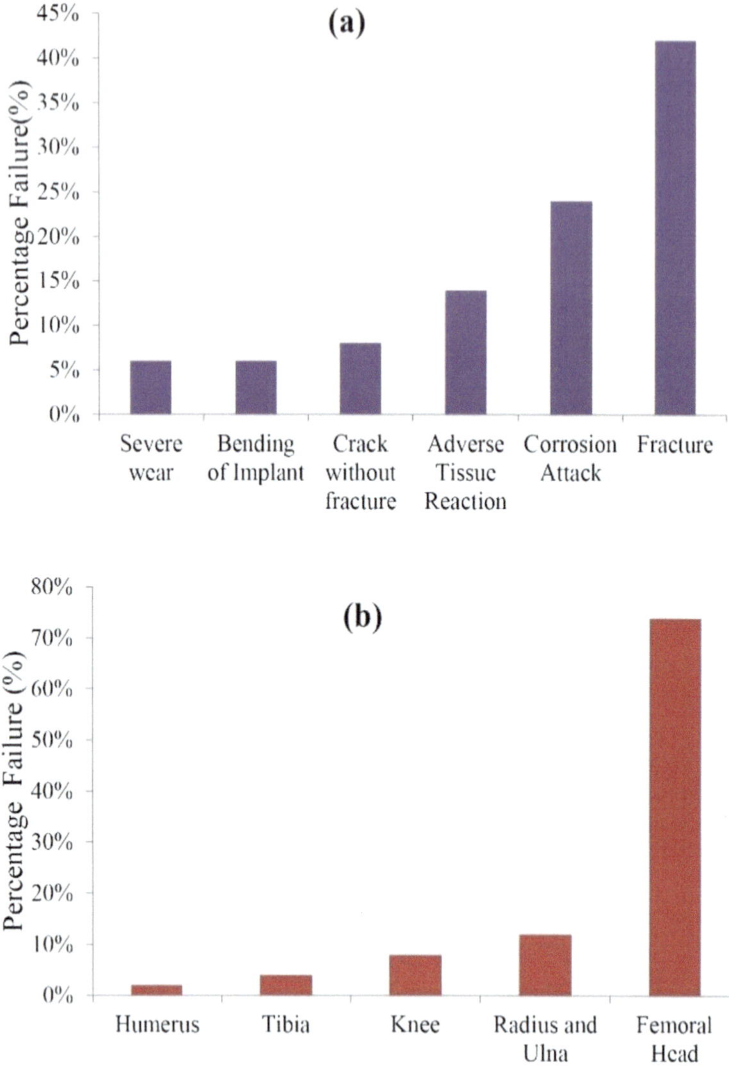

Fig. 2.2 **a** Various reasons for stainless steel implant failures; **b** percentage stainless steel implant failure in different anatomical areas

biocompatibility, and hemocompatibility of the stainless steel. This advancement underscores the importance of electrolyte composition in achieving optimal surface characteristics for biomedical materials.

Synthetic hydroxyapatite (HAp) has emerged as a prominent bioactive coating in biomedical applications, primarily due to its chemical composition, which closely resembles that of natural bone mineral. This similarity is crucial for promoting osteoconductivity and facilitating bone integration. However, one significant drawback of coatings produced via the sol–gel method is their susceptibility to microcracking. These microcracks can compromise the structural integrity of the coating and weaken its adhesion to the underlying substrate, which is essential for long-term performance in biological environments [9]. To combat the issue of microcracking and improve mechanical properties, researchers have increasingly turned to composite coatings. For example, Karamian et al. [14] developed HAp/zirconia composite coatings on 316L stainless steel, a material commonly used in medical implants. Their findings confirmed that the incorporation of zirconia enhanced the mechanical strength and biological performance of the coatings, providing better support for osseointegration, the process by which bone forms around the implant. Figure 2.3 displays the results of X-ray diffraction (XRD) and scanning electron microscopy (SEM) analyses of the NHA/zirconium-coated samples, illustrating the structural and morphological characteristics of the composite layers.

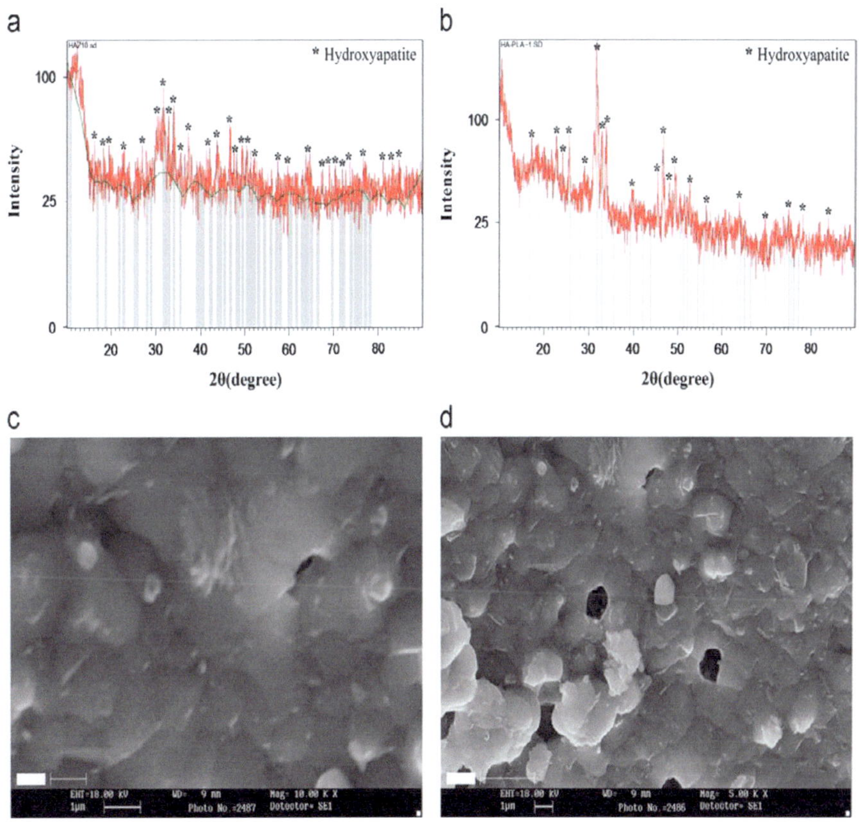

Fig. 2.3 XRD patterns of **a** NHA 0% zircon and **b** NHA 10% zircon coatings on 316L stainless steel. SEM micrographs of **c** NHA 0% zircon and **d** NHA 10% zircon coatings on 316L stainless steel. Reproduced with permission from Elsevier [14]

Zhang et al. [15] conducted a comprehensive study on the adhesion behavior of MC3T3-E1 osteoblast cells on 316L stainless steel surfaces following various surface treatments, including polishing, aluminum oxide blasting, and hydroxyapatite (HAp) coating. Their research revealed that surfaces treated to be rougher and coated with HAp significantly enhanced cell attachment and improved cell morphology when compared to the smoother polished surfaces. This suggests that the physical characteristics of the surface play a crucial role in supporting cellular functions. In a separate study, Zhong et al. [16] utilized atomic layer deposition (ALD) to create a nanometric (10 nm thick) film of aluminum oxide (Al_2O_3) on 316L stainless steel. The application of this thin film resulted in a marked improvement in the surface's hydrophilicity, which is the tendency of a surface to attract water, ultimately leading to better cellular interface characteristics. The enhanced hydrophilicity contributes to improved interactions between the material and biological entities, particularly in biomedical applications. Additionally, Al_2O_3 coatings were found to improve the quality and adhesion of polymer layers on drug-eluting stents (DES), indicating that these coatings could enhance the efficacy and stability of stent materials in a clinical setting. Chang et al. [17] explored the deposition of copper aluminum oxide ($CuAlO_2$) films on 316L stainless steel using radio frequency (RF) magnetron sputtering. Their findings highlighted that the presence of the $CuAlO_2$ layer not only increased the surface hardness of the stainless steel but also bolstered its corrosion resistance. The enhanced hardness is particularly important for applications requiring durable materials, while corrosion resistance is crucial for ensuring longevity and reliability in various environments, especially in medical implants and devices. Overall, these studies underscore the significant impact of surface modifications on the performance of 316L stainless steel in biomedical applications.

Kheirkhah et al. [18] conducted a study on the application of nanostructured forsterite (Mg_2SiO_4) coatings to enhance the surface properties of 316L stainless steel, a material commonly used in biomedical applications. Their research demonstrated that the forsterite-coated specimens exhibited markedly improved corrosion resistance compared to the uncoated samples, which is crucial for longevity and reliability in clinical settings. Additionally, the forsterite coatings significantly enhanced in-vitro bioactivity, suggesting that they may promote better cellular interactions and tissue integration, thereby improving the overall efficacy of stainless steel implants. In a related study, Wang et al. [19] explored the deposition of zirconium carbonitride coatings on 316L austenitic stainless steel. Their findings indicated that these coatings not only enhanced the corrosion resistance of the substrate but also provided important mechanical benefits. The zirconium carbonitride layers, particularly those fabricated at elevated temperatures, were shown to effectively reduce surface roughness and surface energy. This reduction is significant because it can lead to improved blood compatibility, which is essential for materials used in medical implants. Enhanced blood compatibility means a lower risk of thrombosis and better integration with biological tissues, which are critical factors for successful medical implant performance.

Balla et al. [20] utilized Laser Engineered Net Shaping (LENS™) technology to effectively create a coating of bioactive hydroxyapatite (HAp) on the surfaces of 316L stainless steel, a commonly used biomaterial due to its excellent corrosion resistance and mechanical properties. Their research revealed that as the laser energy input was increased, the thickness of the HAp coating also increased. However, this enhancement in coating thickness came with a trade-off, resulting in a reduction of surface hardness. This finding suggests a critical need to balance coating thickness and surface hardness to optimize the performance of surface-modified implants. In another comprehensive study, Bagherifard et al. [21] explored the effects of severe shot peening as a surface treatment technique for AISI 316L stainless steel. Their experiments showed significant improvements in various mechanical attributes. Specifically, the shot peening process led to grain refinement, which is essential for enhancing the material's strength and fatigue resistance. Additionally, they observed improvements in surface roughness and topography, contributing to better interfacial adhesion with biological tissues. The treatment also positively affected wettability and the distribution of residual stresses within the material, which is crucial for the durability and lifespan of implants. Remarkably, this approach not only improved the mechanical properties but also enhanced the biocompatibility of the material, thereby reducing the likelihood of implant loosening or migration within the body. Such advancements highlight the importance of surface treatment techniques in the development and performance of orthopedic implants.

2.2 Magnesium

Biodegradable materials, particularly magnesium and its alloys, have increasingly drawn interest for their potential applications in orthopedic and cardiovascular fields. This is primarily due to their impressive mechanical strength, which makes them suitable for load-bearing implants, and their favorable thermal properties, which can aid in maintaining biological compatibility within the body. However, a significant challenge in using magnesium-based components for medical implants is the formation of an unstable or incomplete oxide layer on their surface. This oxide layer is crucial because it protects the underlying metal from corrosion. When this protective layer is compromised, corrosion accelerates, leading to the premature degradation of the implant material [22]. Another critical issue associated with the corrosion of magnesium alloys is the uncontrolled generation of hydrogen gas. During the corrosion process, hydrogen can be released, and if this release occurs too rapidly, it can lead to the accumulation of gas pockets. These pockets can obstruct blood flow, potentially resulting in serious physiological complications, including ischemia or tissue necrosis [23]. To mitigate these challenges and enhance the corrosion resistance of magnesium and its alloys, researchers have proposed two primary strategies. The first involves altering the alloy's composition and refining its microstructure. This includes manipulation of grain size, which can improve mechanical properties and corrosion resistance by refining the material's microstructure at the atomic level [24, 25]. The second strategy focuses on the application of surface treatments or protective coatings. These coatings can act as barriers to corrosion, preventing direct contact between the magnesium and the bodily fluids, thereby slowing down the corrosion rate and controlling hydrogen gas release [26]. Through these innovative approaches, researchers aim to unlock the full potential of magnesium-based implants, ensuring they are both safe and effective for use in medical applications.

Razavi et al. [27] conducted a study aimed at enhancing the in-vitro bioactivity and corrosion resistance of biodegradable magnesium alloys, which are of significant interest in biomedical applications such as implants. Their approach combined micro-arc oxidation (MAO) and electrophoretic deposition (EPD) to form protective coatings on the magnesium surfaces. The MAO process creates a hardened layer on the metal by forming an oxide on its surface, while EPD allows for the uniform deposition of materials. This innovative technique resulted in the formation of nanostructured coatings composed of akermanite and diopside ($CaMgSi_2O_6$), both of which are known to exhibit favorable biocompatibility and bioactivity. These coatings effectively shielded the underlying magnesium from aggressive corrosive environments, thus prolonging the lifespan of the biodegradable implants. Similarly, Chen et al. [28] explored a conversion coating method that utilized strontium phosphate (SrP) to address the early-stage degradation of magnesium, which can occur due to exposure to physiological conditions. They prepared a coating solution consisting of 0.1 M strontium and 0.06 M phosphate ions, which was heated to 80 °C in a minimum essential medium (MEM) to stimulate the reaction. This controlled environment facilitated the formation of a protective layer of strontium apatite (SrAP) on the magnesium surface. The resultant SrAP layer significantly improved the corrosion resistance of magnesium implants by providing a stable barrier against corrosive agents. Additionally, the coating helped to alleviate the cytotoxic effects associated with the hydrogen gas released during magnesium degradation, thereby enhancing the overall safety and efficacy of magnesium-based implants in clinical settings.

In an exploratory study conducted by Kannan [29], the effectiveness of calcium phosphate films applied to magnesium alloys was evaluated through various electrochemical techniques. Two distinct coating methods were examined: the pulse-potential method and the constant-potential method. The results revealed that the pulse-potential method provided significantly superior corrosion protection, demonstrating a polarization resistance that was three times greater than that achieved with the constant-potential coating. This finding highlights the advantages of employing pulse-potential techniques to enhance the longevity and stability of magnesium alloys in corrosive environments. Figure 2.4 illustrates the surface morphology of the coated alloys obtained via both methods, showcasing the structural differences introduced by each coating technique. Lu [30] conducted a separate investigation that focused on the application of β-tricalcium phosphate (CaP) coatings, which were formed through chemical reactions in simulated Hank's solution, a commonly used in-vitro environment for studying biological processes. The resulting CaP coatings were found to significantly enhance the bioactivity of the magnesium substrates, effectively reduce the degradation rate, and improve corrosion resistance. These properties are particularly beneficial for biomedical applications, such as in implants, where stability and biocompatibility are crucial. In a further advancement of this research, Lu et al. [31] incorporated strontium into the CaP coating to develop a novel Ca–Sr–P layer on

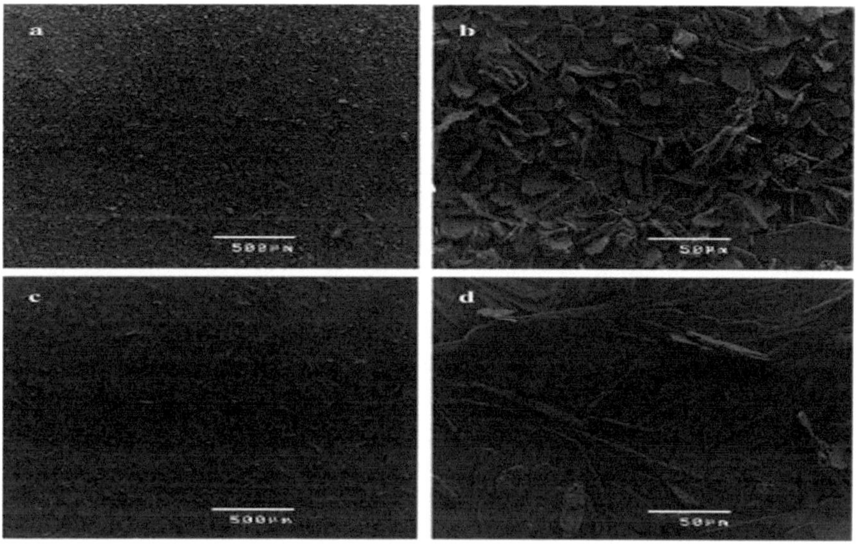

Fig. 2.4 SEM of the calcium phosphate coated AZ91 magnesium alloy using different coating methods: **a**, **b** randomly dispersed coating via constant-potential and **c**, **d** compact coating via the pulse-potential method. Reproduced with permission from Elsevier [29]

pure magnesium substrates. This modification resulted in a coating with a uniform and refined microstructure, which not only provided enhanced surface protection and corrosion resistance but also contributed to improved biocompatibility of the implant material. By integrating strontium, a trace element known to promote bone health, into the coating, the research aimed to foster better integration of the implant with the surrounding biological tissue, thus potentially improving clinical outcomes for patients.

Mahapatro et al. [32] conducted a comprehensive review on the application of nanostructured self-assembled monolayers (SAMs) for the surface modification of magnesium and its alloys. Their research highlighted the potential of SAMs as an innovative approach to enhance the surface properties of biodegradable magnesium substrates. This enhancement is particularly significant for improving biological interface interactions and cellular responses, which are crucial for applications in biomedical fields such as implants and drug delivery systems. In a related study, White et al. [33] employed the plasma electrolytic oxidation (PEO) technique to improve the mechanical properties of the AZ31 magnesium alloy, a commonly used material in various engineering applications due to its lightweight and strength. They systematically evaluated the effects of three distinct electrolyte formulations, each varying in concentrations of NaOH, Na_2SiO_3, KF, and NaH_2PO_4. Their findings revealed that the PEO coating formulated with potassium fluoride (KF) led to a remarkable enhancement in several key properties of the alloy. Specifically, this treatment significantly increased the corrosion resistance, wear resistance, surface hardness, and elastic modulus of the AZ31 magnesium substrate when compared to its untreated state. These advancements underscore the effectiveness of the PEO technique in optimizing the performance and longevity of magnesium alloys in challenging environments.

2.3 Titanium

Titanium and its alloys are increasingly recognized as some of the most important metallic biomaterials utilized in the fields of orthopedics, dentistry, and other critical biomedical applications. This popularity can be attributed to their remarkable mechanical and biological properties, which include excellent strength-to-weight ratios, corrosion resistance, and biocompatibility. A pivotal study indicates that more than 1000 tonnes, equivalent to approximately 2.2 million individual titanium-based devices, are implanted in patients globally each year, underscoring the material's extensive use in healthcare [34]. In their research, Ucar and Balo [35] conducted a thorough comparative analysis of various mechanical parameters, including Young's modulus, compressive strength, yield strength, and tensile strength, across different biomaterials. Their comprehensive findings revealed that titanium demonstrates superior mechanical performance in all evaluated factors. As a result, titanium has become one of the most favored materials for the fabrication of implants, providing a reliable and effective solution for medical professionals. This is illustrated in Fig. 2.5, which compares the mechanical properties of titanium with those of other biomaterials, reinforcing its status as a leading choice in biomedical applications.

While titanium and its alloys are known for their lightweight and corrosion-resistant properties, they are often not the first choice for load-bearing applications

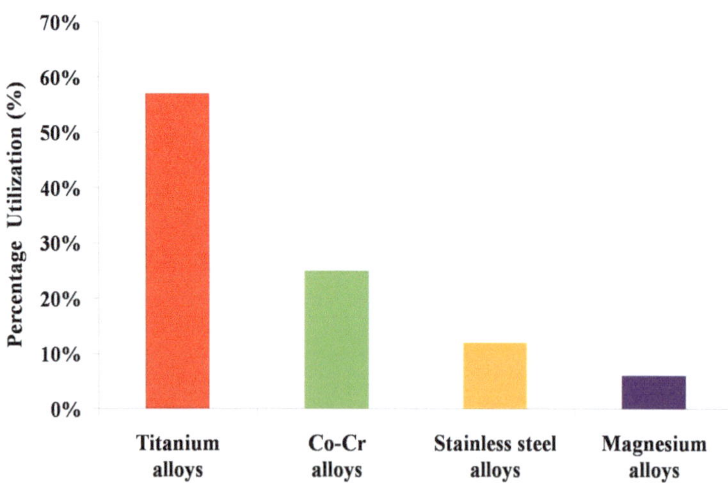

Fig. 2.5 Biomaterials according to priority values

due to their limited tribological performance. This performance limitation is particularly evident in their fatigue strength and wear resistance, which are critical factors in applications where durability and longevity are paramount (Fig. 2.6) [36]. To address these issues, researchers and engineers have developed a range of advanced surface modification techniques aimed at enhancing the surface characteristics of titanium alloys without compromising their inherent bulk properties. These surface treatments can significantly improve wear resistance, fatigue life, and overall performance under demanding conditions. Among the most effective surface modification methods are grit blasting, which creates a roughened surface that can enhance adhesion for coatings; chemical etching, which removes contaminants and can improve surface characteristics at the microscopic level; and titanium plasma spraying, which deposits a protective coating that enhances wear resistance. Additionally, laser processing can be employed to precisely alter surface textures and properties, while electrochemical treatments can lead to improved corrosion resistance and surface hardness [37]. By employing a combination of these methods, engineers can tailor the surface properties of titanium alloys to meet specific application requirements, thus expanding their usability in high-performance and load-bearing environments.

The emergence of allergic reactions linked to Ti–6Al–4V alloys in biomedical applications has spurred researchers to seek alternative titanium-based materials that can mitigate these issues. One promising avenue in this pursuit involves the integration of second-generation beta-phase stabilizers, such as niobium (Nb), tantalum (Ta), and zirconium (Zr). These elements are being used not only to enhance biocompatibility but also to eliminate concerns regarding cytotoxicity, which is critical for materials intended for implantation in the human body. In their groundbreaking work,

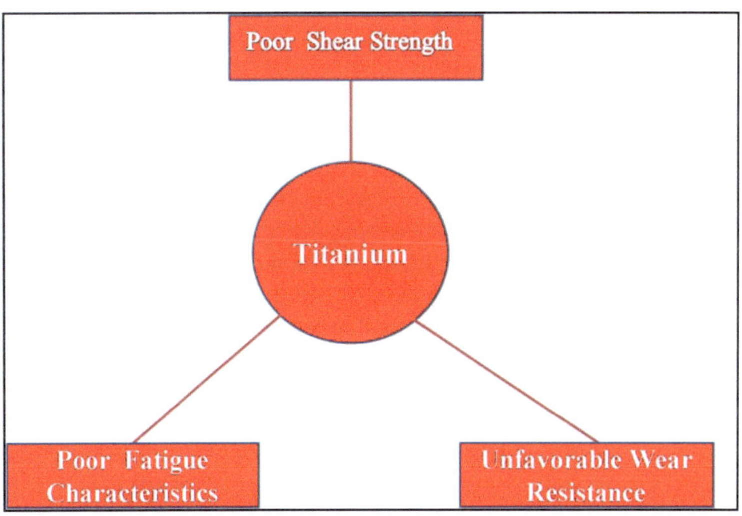

Fig. 2.6 Causes for failure of titanium implant

Kuroda et al. [38] employed a d-electron alloy design methodology to develop innovative beta-type titanium alloys that are composed entirely of non-toxic elements. Their research focused on synthesizing alloys containing Nb, Ta, Zr, molybdenum (Mo), and tin (Sn), which are known for their positive biological interactions. The results of their study revealed that the newly formulated Ti–29Nb–13Ta–4.6Zr alloy demonstrated tensile strength and elongation properties that were comparable to or superior to those of conventional titanium alloys. Additionally, its Young's modulus was found to be significantly closer to that of natural bone. This property is particularly important because it promotes better integration of the implant with surrounding bone tissue and minimizes the risk of stress shielding, a condition where the bone weakens due to decreased mechanical loading.

Similarly, Taddei et al. [39] harnessed powder metallurgy techniques to fabricate a porous Ti–35Nb–7Zr–5Ta alloy. This process involves blending elemental powders of Nb, Ta, Zr, and Ti to create a microstructure that is ideally suited for orthopedic implants. The mechanical evaluations of this alloy highlighted its high strength, favorable porosity, and outstanding interfacial bonding capabilities. These features contribute to its viability as a candidate for a range of biomedical applications, particularly in load-bearing contexts where durability and compatibility are essential. Furthermore, Niinomi [40] conducted a comprehensive investigation into the mechanical reliability of titanium alloys used in medical and dental implants under simulated physiological conditions. This study took into account the dynamic and complex environment within the human body. The results indicated that crucial properties such as crack propagation rate, Vickers hardness, and fracture toughness remained stable over time, affirming the long-term reliability and performance of these advanced materials in clinical settings. This stability is vital for ensuring the safety and effectiveness of implants, ultimately leading to improved patient outcomes.

To improve the surface characteristics of titanium implants, Liu et al. [41] introduced innovative plasma-based surface modification techniques, specifically plasma spraying and plasma immersion ion implantation and deposition (PIII-D). Their research revealed that PIII-D not only provided superior interfacial bonding between the coating and the titanium substrate but also outperformed traditional plasma spraying methods in terms of adhesion strength. Furthermore, by incorporating bioactive elements such as calcium, phosphorus, and sodium directly into the surface layer using PIII-D, they significantly enhanced the biocompatibility and bioactivity of the titanium implants, which is crucial for successful integration into biological tissues. In addition to plasma-based techniques, laser-based technologies have emerged as powerful tools for precise surface treatment of titanium implants. Trtica et al. [42] demonstrated the effectiveness of using Nd: YAG lasers for modifying the surface topography of titanium implants. Their findings showed that the laser treatment resulted in enhanced morphology and surface roughness, both of which are critical for improving bio-integration with the surrounding bone tissue. Similarly, Braga et al. [43] employed an Nd: YVO_4 laser to treat titanium dental implants, achieving precise modifications to the titanium oxide passivation layer. This targeted enhancement led to improved osseointegration and increased clinical stability of the implants, highlighting the advantages of laser technologies in dental applications.

Additionally, Mendes et al. [44] investigated the synthesis of a low-modulus Ti–27Nb–13Zr alloy through powder metallurgy and subjected the resulting samples to a biomimetic treatment in simulated body fluid (SBF), which is rich in calcium and phosphate ions. This treatment effectively induced the formation of an appetite-promoting layer on the alloy surface, which is essential for enhancing biological interactions. Subsequent evaluations indicated significant improvements in microhardness and elastic modulus, suggesting that this alloy possesses favorable mechanical properties for orthopedic and dental applications. The combination of these properties makes it a promising candidate for use in environments requiring both strength and biocompatibility.

2.4 Cobalt-Chromium

Cobalt-based alloys have increasingly gained recognition as a leading choice for biomedical applications due to their remarkable combination of properties. These materials are characterized by excellent corrosion resistance, which prevents degradation in the harsh environments of the human body; high mechanical strength, providing durability; reliable wear resistance, crucial for long-lasting performance; and favorable biocompatibility, ensuring they do not provoke adverse reactions from the surrounding tissues [45]. These alloys are extensively utilized in various orthopedic procedures and dental prosthetics. They play a critical role in joint replacements, where they are used to create prosthetic components that can withstand the significant stresses experienced in load-bearing joints. Similarly, in dental applications, cobalt-chromium alloys are favored for dental implants, providing a stable foundation for artificial teeth. One of the standout features of Co–Cr alloys is their strong osseointegration capabilities. This property ensures a stable and functional interface between the implant surface and the surrounding bone and soft tissue, which is crucial for the long-term success of any implant. Strong osseointegration minimizes the risk of implant failure and enhances overall functionality and comfort for the patient [46]. In a comparative study conducted by Beake and Liskiewicz [47], the wear properties of three different alloys, Ti–6Al–4V, 316L stainless steel, and Co–Cr, were evaluated. The results showed that Co–Cr alloys outperformed the other materials in terms of wear resistance, highlighting their superior durability in applications where friction and mechanical wear are significant concerns. This reinforces the appeal of cobalt-based alloys in the development of reliable and effective biomedical devices.

Supporting evidence from various studies underscores the significant advantages of cobalt-chromium (Co–Cr) alloys, particularly in orthopedic applications such as hip joint prostheses. A substantial percentage of these prostheses are constructed from Co–Cr alloys due to their remarkable combination of high strength, excellent

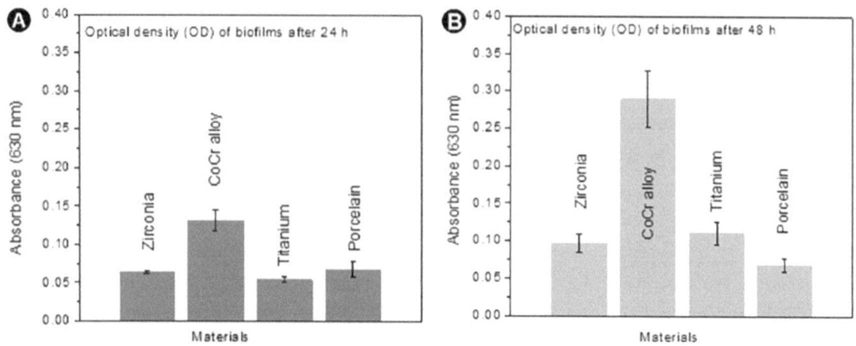

Fig. 2.7 Optical density of the biofilm growth on the various materials. Reproduced under license CC-BY-4.0 [49]

ductility, and impressive resistance to both wear and corrosion. These mechanical properties ensure that the implants can withstand the stresses and strains of daily movement, ultimately increasing their longevity and functionality [48]. In addition to their mechanical advantages, Co–Cr alloys have demonstrated a noteworthy capability to foster the formation of biocompatible surface films. These films are essential as they enhance the integration of the implant with the body, promoting healing and reducing the risk of rejection. Compared to many other metallic implant materials, Co–Cr alloys have shown superior performance in this regard, which is a crucial factor contributing to their widespread clinical success [49]. A visual representation of these advantages can be found in Fig. 2.7, which illustrates the benefits of Co–Cr alloys in orthopedic applications.

Co–Cr alloys are extensively utilized in biomedical applications, particularly in orthopedic implants, due to their favorable mechanical properties and resistance to wear. However, they present critical biocompatibility concerns stemming from the release of metal ions into the surrounding tissues and bodily fluids. Studies have shown that elevated concentrations of cobalt and chromium ions can be detected in synovial fluid and peripheral blood following the implantation of these alloys, raising significant toxicity concerns for patients. This ion release is primarily due to bio-corrosion, a complex process that occurs over time as the metal interfaces with the physiological environment, leading to the degradation of the material [50]. Bio-corrosion poses a considerable challenge for the long-term performance and safety of orthopedic implants, necessitating effective solutions to enhance the stability and biocompatibility of Co–Cr alloys [51]. To tackle this problem, surface engineering has emerged as a promising strategy to improve the corrosion resistance of these alloys. For instance, Metikos-Hukovic et al. [52] demonstrated the effectiveness of creating a stable passive oxide layer on Co–Cr–Mo alloys when immersed in Hank's solution. This oxide layer significantly improved both corrosion resistance and biocompatibility, suggesting that proper surface modification can mitigate harmful ion release. Further advancements in this field were achieved by Liu et al. [53], who employed innovative plasma surface alloying techniques. By introducing nitrogen and carbon into the surface of Co–Cr alloys through methods such as plasma nitriding and carbonitriding, they successfully enhanced the metallurgical and mechanical properties of the alloys, as well as their resistance to corrosion and wear. This approach not only improves the longevity of the implants but also helps to protect the surrounding biological tissues. Moreover, Díaz et al. [54] explored the use of plasma immersion ion implantation as a strategy to minimize metal ion release from Co–Cr substrates. Their treatment facilitated the formation of a thick and stable chromium oxide layer, which is known to enhance wear resistance and further reduce the leaching of harmful ions into the body. These advances in surface engineering highlight the potential for improving the safety and effectiveness of Co–Cr alloys in medical applications, addressing the critical issue of biocompatibility while ensuring the long-term success of orthopedic implants.

Surface modification utilizing self-assembled monolayers (SAMs) has emerged as a significant focus in materials science, particularly for biomedical applications. In their study, Mani et al. [55] investigated the use of octadecyl trichlorosilane (OTS) SAMs on cobalt-chromium (Co–Cr) alloys, aiming to enhance the surface stability and performance of these materials in medical environments. The OTS SAMs create a hydrophobic layer that potentially reduces protein adsorption and cellular adhesion, which are crucial factors in the longevity and effectiveness of biomedical implants. Similarly, Bhure et al. [56] contributed to this field by developing and characterizing octadecyl phosphonic acid (ODPA)-based SAMs on Co–Cr alloy surfaces. Their research highlighted the advantageous properties of these coatings, which not only improve surface chemistry but also significantly enhance stability. The ODPA SAMs facilitate biocompatibility, making them promising candidates for various biomedical implants, including orthopedic and dental applications. In another notable advancement, Zhou et al. [57] and their research team introduced cobalt-based bulk metallic glasses (BMGs) as cutting-edge materials for biomedical uses. Their investigations revealed that specific compositions, particularly $Cr_{10}Mo_{10}$, exhibited exceptional corrosion resistance and biocompatibility when compared to traditional materials like 316L stainless steel. This characteristic is vital for implants, as it not only prolongs their lifespan but also minimizes the risk of adverse biological reactions. Additionally, these BMGs show a significant reduction in biofouling, further enhancing their suitability for long-term applications within the human body. Overall, the incorporation of SAMs and BMGs presents exciting opportunities for advancements in the design and performance of biomedical implants.

Yang et al. [58] conducted a comprehensive investigation into Ni–Co–Cr alloys, revealing that the precise adjustment of cobalt and chromium ratios significantly influenced the alloy's elastic properties as well as its solution-strengthening behavior. This adjustment plays a crucial role in optimizing the mechanical performance of the alloys under various conditions. In addition, corrosion-wear studies on Co–Cr–W alloys exposed to liquid zinc environments demonstrated that degradation processes were accelerated due to the corrosion of eutectic phases combined with the high temperatures of the zinc [59]. These findings underscore the importance of material composition and environmental factors in applications involving high-temperature corrosion resistance. Efforts to enhance the mechanical durability of Co–Cr–Mo alloys have been actively pursued through various reinforcement techniques. Sahasrabudhe et al. [60] utilized Laser Engineered Net Shaping (LENS™) technology to incorporate calcium phosphate (CaP) into the Co–Cr–Mo matrix. This innovative approach not only led to a marked improvement in wear resistance, making the alloys more suitable for demanding applications, but it also effectively reduced the leaching of metal ions, addressing concerns over biocompatibility in biomedical applications.

Furthermore, Nova et al. [61] discovered that the inclusion of niobium in Co–Cr–Mo alloys resulted in significant improvements in surface hardness and wear resistance, which are critical properties for applications subjected to high friction and wear. This enhancement was clearly illustrated in Fig. 2.8, emphasizing the potential for tailored material properties through strategic alloying. Chiba et al. [62] highlighted the critical influence of manufacturing processes on the wear behavior of Co–Cr–Mo alloys. Their research demonstrated that forged variants of these alloys exhibited superior wear resistance compared to their cast counterparts, particularly those with high carbon content. This finding suggests that the processing methods employed during fabrication can profoundly affect the physical and mechanical properties of the final product, thereby influencing its performance in practical applications. Overall, these studies illustrate the intricate relationships between composition, processing, and performance in advanced alloy systems.

Bose et al. [63] conducted an in-depth exploration of various Additive Manufacturing (AM) techniques, focusing on their potential to enhance the surface characteristics of biomaterials. Their findings indicated that AM processes can lead to significant improvements in the wear and abrasion resistance of cobalt-based materials, which are commonly used in biomedical applications due to their favorable mechanical properties and biocompatibility. In a related investigation, Cetiner et al. [64] reported that the application of a titanium dioxide (TiO_2) coating on cobalt-chromium (Co–Cr) alloys not only augmented their surface wear resistance but also positively affected their biological activity. This enhancement can be attributed to the TiO_2 coating, which is known for its biocompatibility and ability to promote cell adhesion. To provide a clearer overview, a comprehensive summary of the various surface modification techniques applied to metallic biomaterials is compiled in Table 2.1, highlighting the effectiveness and potential applications of these methods in improving the performance of materials used in medical implants and devices.

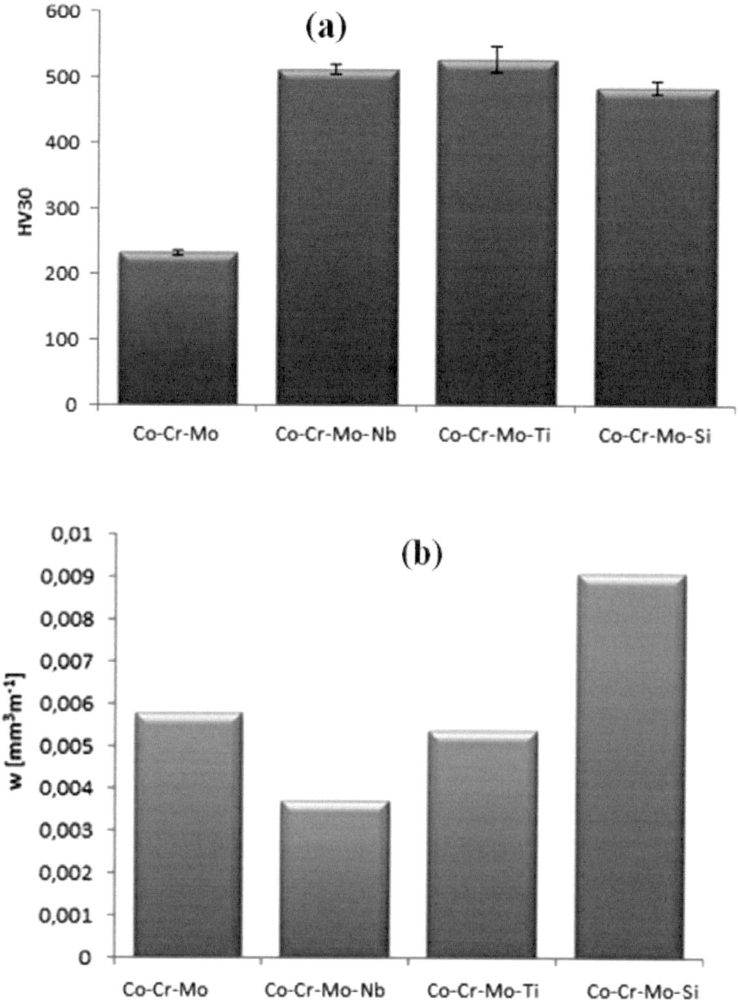

Fig. 2.8 Co–Cr alloy composition versus **a** hardness; **b** wear rate. Reproduced under license CC-BY-4.0 [61]

Table 2.1 Literature summary of surface modification of different materials by various effectual techniques

Material	Coating	Method	References
Stainless steel	Hydroxyapatite	Water-based sol–gel	[9]
	Non acid ionic liquid	Electrochemical pretreatment	[11]
	Electrochemical polishing	Chemical surface treatment	[12]
	Electrochemically polishing	Chemical surface treatment	[13]
	Hydroxyapatite/zircon nano-biocomposite	Plasma spray method	[14]
	Hydroxyapatite, aluminum oxide blasting, polishing	Plasma spraying	[15]
	Al_2O_3	Atomic layer deposition	[16]
	$CuAlO_2$	Radiofrequency magnetron sputtering method	[17]
	Mg_2SiO_4	Sol–gel dip	[18]
	Zirconium carbonitride	Radiofrequency magnetron sputtering method	[19]
	Hydroxyapatite	LENS	[20]
	Uncoated	Severe shot peening	[21]
Magnesium	Nanostructured diopside, nanostructured akermanite	Micro arc oxidation with electrophoretic deposition	[27]
	Strontium phosphate	Minimum essential medium	[28]
	Calcium phosphate	Pulse potential method	[29]
	Calcium phosphate and calcium phosphate with strontium	Hank's solution	[30, 31]
	NaOH, Na_2SiO_3, KF and NaH_2PO_4	Plasma electrolytic oxidation	[32]
Titanium	Nb, Ta, Zr, Mo, Sn powders	D-electron alloy design method	[38]
	Nb, Ta, Zr, Ti powders	Blended element method	[39]
	(a) Hydroxyapatite (b) Calcium silicate (c) Phosphorous powders (d) Sodium powders	Plasma spraying and plasma immersion ion (PIII-D)	[41]
	Uncoated	Nd: YAG laser	[42]
	Uncoated	Nd: YVO_4 laser	[43]
	Biomimetic	Powder metallurgy	[44]
Cobalt-chromium (Co–Cr)	Passive oxide film	Hank's solution	[52]
	Nitrogen and carbon powder	Plasma surface alloying method	[53]

(continued)

Table 2.1 (continued)

Material	Coating	Method	References
	Chromium oxide	PIII	[54]
	Self-assembled monolayers	Octadecyltrichlorosilane (OTS)	[55]
	Self-assembled monolayers	Octadecyl phosphonic (ODPA)	[56]
	Uncoated	Co-based BMGs	[57]
	Uncoated	Varying the amount of Co and Cr in Ni–Co–Cr alloys	[58]
	Calcium phosphate (CaP)	Laser engineered net shaping (LENS™)	[60]
	Uncoated	Adding Nb in Co–Cr–Mo alloy	[61]
	Uncoated	Additive manufacturing (AM)	[63]
	Titanium oxide	Cold spray and thermal oxidation	[64]

2.5 Conclusions

This chapter provides an in-depth analysis of surface modification strategies for key metallic biomaterials utilized in biomedical implants, specifically focusing on stainless steel, magnesium, titanium, and cobalt-chromium alloys. Each of these materials presents distinct challenges that impact their performance in medical applications. For instance, stainless steel is often susceptible to corrosion in biological environments. Magnesium has issues with rapid degradation in bodily fluids; titanium, while biocompatible, can experience wear over time, and cobalt-chromium, although highly durable, may pose biocompatibility concerns. To address these challenges, various surface engineering techniques have been developed to enhance the properties of these materials. Sol–gel coatings, for example, create a thin, protective layer that improves corrosion resistance while also being biocompatible. Laser treatments can modify the surface microstructure of implants, enhance their mechanical strength, and promote better bone integration. Plasma-based processes, such as plasma spraying or plasma nitriding, can significantly improve wear resistance and fatigue strength. These advancements in surface modification are critical for extending the lifespan of implants and ensuring their seamless integration with human tissue. By improving these interactions, we can reduce the risk of implant failure and the need for revision surgeries. Continued research in this field is essential, particularly into the development of multifunctional surfaces that can simultaneously address multiple challenges, such as enhancing biocompatibility, corrosion resistance, and mechanical properties. This research will play a pivotal role in paving the way for the next generation of medical implants, which are expected to be more effective in supporting patient outcomes.

References

1. Geanta V, Voiculescu I, Stefanoiu R, Rusu ER (2014) Stainless steels with biocompatible properties for medical devices. Key Eng Mater 583:9–15
2. Piehler HR (1985) Pluralistic medical device risk management: standards, regulation, and litigation. In: Fraker AC, Griffin CD (eds) Corrosion and degradation of implant materials: second symposium. ASTM International, Pennsylvania, pp 1–10
3. Zhang F, Kang ET, Neoh KG, Wang P, Tan KL (2001) Surface modification of stainless steel by grafting of poly(ethylene glycol) for reduction in protein adsorption. Biomaterials 22(12):1541–1548
4. Lewis AL, Tolhurst LA, Stratford PW (2002) Analysis of a phosphorylcholine-based polymer coating on a coronary stent pre- and post-implantation. Biomaterials 23(7):1697–1706
5. Hanawa T (2003) Reconstruction and regeneration of surface oxide film on metallic materials in biological environments. Corros Rev 21:161–181
6. Sivakumar M, Kumar Dhanadurai KS, Rajeswari S, Thulasiraman V (1995) Failures in stainless steel orthopaedic implant devices: a survey. J Mater Sci Lett 14(5):351–354
7. Kang CK, Lee YS (2007) The surface modification of stainless steel and the correlation between the surface properties and protein adsorption. J Mater Sci Mater Med 18(7):1389–1398
8. Thakur A, Kumar A, Kaya S, Marzouki R, Zhang F, Guo L (2022) Recent advancements in surface modification, characterization and functionalization for enhancing the biocompatibility and corrosion resistance of biomedical implants. Coatings 12(10):1459
9. Liu DM, Yang Q, Troczynski T (2002) Sol–gel hydroxyapatite coatings on stainless steel substrates. Biomaterials 23(3):691–698
10. Shih CC, Shih CM, Su YY, Su LHJ, Chang MS, Lin SJ (2004) Effect of surface oxide properties on corrosion resistance of 316L stainless steel for biomedical applications. Corros Sci 46(2):427–441
11. Abdel-Fattah TM, Loftis D, Mahapatro A (2011) Nanosized controlled surface pretreatment of biometallic alloy 316L stainless steel. J Biomed Nanotechnol 7(6):794–800
12. Latifi A, Imani M, Khorasani MT, Joupari MD (2013) Electrochemical and chemical methods for improving surface characteristics of 316L stainless steel for biomedical applications. Surf Coat Technol 221:1–12
13. Habibzadeh S, Li L, Shum-Tim D, Davis EC, Omanovic S (2014) Electrochemical polishing as a 316L stainless steel surface treatment method: towards the improvement of biocompatibility. Corros Sci 87:89–100
14. Karamian E, Motamedi MRK, Khandan A, Soltani P, Maghsoudi S (2014) An in vitro evaluation of novel NHA/zircon plasma coating on 316L stainless steel dental implant. Prog Nat Sci Mater Int 24(2):150–156
15. Zhang H, Han J, Sun Y, Huang Y, Zhou M (2015) MC3T3-E1 cell response to stainless steel 316L with different surface treatments. Mater Sci Eng C 56:22–29
16. Zhong Q, Yan J, Qian X, Zhang T, Zhang Z, Li A (2014) Atomic layer deposition enhanced grafting of phosphorylcholine on stainless steel for intravascular stents. Colloids Surf B 121:238–247
17. Chang SH, Chen JZ, Hsiao SH, Lin GW (2014) Nanohardness, corrosion and protein adsorption properties of $CuAlO_2$ films deposited on 316L stainless steel for biomedical applications. Appl Surf Sci 289:455–461

18. Kheirkhah M, Fathi M, Salimijazi HR, Razavi M (2015) Surface modification of stainless steel implants using nanostructured forsterite (Mg_2SiO_4) coating for biomaterial applications. Surf Coat Technol 276:580–586
19. Wang L, Zhao X, Ding MH, Zheng H, Zhang HS, Zhang B, Li XQ, Wu GY (2015) Surface modification of biomedical AISI 316L stainless steel with zirconium carbonitride coatings. Appl Surf Sci 340:113–119
20. Balla VK, Das M, Bose S, Ram GJ, Manna I (2013) Laser surface modification of 316 L stainless steel with bioactive hydroxyapatite. Mater Sci Eng C 33(8):4594–4598
21. Bagherifard S, Slawik S, Fernández-Pariente I, Pauly C, Mücklich F, Guagliano M (2016) Nanoscale surface modification of AISI 316L stainless steel by severe shot peening. Mater Des 102:68–77
22. Liu N, Huang WM (2006) DSC study on temperature memory effect of NiTi shape memory alloy. Trans Nonferrous Met Soc China 16:s37–s41
23. Hornberger H, Virtanen S, Boccaccini AR (2012) Biomedical coatings on magnesium alloys—a review. Acta Biomater 8(7):2442–2455
24. Wang H, Estrin Y, Zúberova Z (2008) Bio-corrosion of a magnesium alloy with different processing histories. Mater Lett 62(16):2476–2479
25. Birbilis N, Zhang MX, Estrin Y (2008) Surface grain size effects on the corrosion of magnesium. Key Eng Mater 384:229–240
26. Gray J, Luan B (2002) Protective coatings on magnesium and its alloys—a critical review. J Alloys Compd 336(1–2):88–113
27. Razavi M, Fathi M, Savabi O, Razavi SM, Beni BH, Vashaee D, Tayebi L (2014) Controlling the degradation rate of bioactive magnesium implants by electrophoretic deposition of akermanite coating. Ceram Int 40(3):3865–3872
28. Chen XB, Nisbet DR, Li RW, Smith PN, Abbott TB, Easton MA, Zhang DH, Birbilis N (2014) Controlling initial biodegradation of magnesium by a biocompatible strontium phosphate conversion coating. Acta Biomater 10(3):1463–1474
29. Kannan MB (2012) Enhancing the performance of calcium phosphate coating on a magnesium alloy for bioimplant applications. Mater Lett 76:109–112
30. Lu Y, Tan L, Xiang H, Zhang B, Yang K, Li Y (2012) Fabrication and characterization of Ca–Mg–P containing coating on pure magnesium. J Mater Sci Technol 28(7):636–641
31. Lu Y, Tan L, Zhang B, Lin J, Yang K (2014) Synthesis and characterization of Ca–Sr–P coating on pure magnesium for biomedical application. Ceram Int 40(3):4559–4565
32. Mahapatro A, Matos Negron TD, Gomes AS (2016) Nanostructured self assembled monolayers on magnesium for improved biological performance. Mater Technol 31(13):818–827
33. White L, Koo Y, Neralla S, Sankar J, Yun Y (2016) Enhanced mechanical properties and increased corrosion resistance of a biodegradable magnesium alloy by plasma electrolytic oxidation (PEO). Mater Sci Eng B 208:39–46
34. Geetha M, Singh AK, Asokamani R, Gogia AK (2009) Ti based biomaterials, the ultimate choice for orthopaedic implants—a review. Prog Mater Sci 54(3):397–425
35. Ucar U, Balo B (2018) Determining of the convenient metal dental implant material in terms of strength properties. Org Med Chem Int J 6(2):555–683
36. Alam MO, Haseeb ASMA (2002) Response of Ti–6Al–4V and Ti–24Al–11Nb alloys to dry sliding wear against hardened steel. Tribol Int 35(6):357–362
37. Vorobyev AY, Guo C (2007) Femtosecond laser structuring of titanium implants. Appl Surf Sci 253(17):7272–7280
38. Kuroda D, Niinomi M, Morinaga M, Kato Y, Yashiro T (1998) Design and mechanical properties of new β type titanium alloys for implant materials. Mater Sci Eng A 243(1–2):244–249
39. Taddei EB, Henriques VAR, Silva CRM, Cairo CAA (2004) Production of new titanium alloy for orthopedic implants. Mater Sci Eng C 24(5):683–687
40. Niinomi M (1998) Mechanical properties of biomedical titanium alloys. Mater Sci Eng A 243:231–236

41. Liu X, Poon RW, Kwok SC, Chu PK, Ding C (2004) Plasma surface modification of titanium for hard tissue replacements. Surf Coat Technol 186(1–2):227–233
42. Trtica M, Gakovic B, Batani D, Desai T, Panjan P, Radak B (2006) Surface modifications of a titanium implant by a picosecond Nd: YAG laser operating at 1064 and 532 nm. Appl Surf Sci 253(5):2551–2556
43. Braga FJ, Marques RF, de A Filho E, Guastaldi AC (2007) Surface modification of Ti dental implants by Nd: YVO_4 laser irradiation. Appl Surf Sci 253(23):9203–9208
44. Mendes MW, Ágreda CG, Bressiani AH, Bressiani JC (2016) A new titanium based alloy Ti–27Nb–13Zr produced by powder metallurgy with biomimetic coating for use as a biomaterial. Mater Sci Eng C 63:671–677
45. Gibson N, Stamm H (2002) The use of alloys in prosthetic devices. In: Business briefing: medical device manufacturing technology, pp 48–51
46. Hyslop DJS, Abdelkader AM, Cox A, Fray DJ (2010) Electrochemical synthesis of a biomedically important Co–Cr alloy. Acta Mater 58(8):3124–3130
47. Beake BD, Liskiewicz TW (2013) Comparison of nano-fretting and nano-scratch tests on biomedical materials. Tribol Int 63:123–131
48. Niinomi M (2002) Recent metallic materials for biomedical applications. Metall Mater Trans A 33(3):477
49. Souza J, Mota RR, Sordi MB, Passoni BB, Benfatti CA, Magini RS (2016) Biofilm formation on different materials used in oral rehabilitation. Braz Dent J 27(2):141–147
50. Posada OM, Tate RJ, Grant MH (2015) Effects of CoCr metal wear debris generated from metal-on-metal hip implants and Co ions on human monocyte-like U937 cells. Toxicol In Vitro 29(2):271–280
51. Sargeant A, Goswami T (2007) Hip implants–paper VI–ion concentrations. Mater Des 28(1):155–171
52. Metikos-Hukovic M, Pilic Z, Babic R, Omanovic D (2006) Influence of alloying elements on the corrosion stability of Co–Cr–Mo implant alloy in Hank's solution. Acta Biomater 2(6):693–700
53. Liu R, Li X, Hu X, Dong H (2013) Surface modification of a medical grade Co–Cr–Mo alloy by low-temperature plasma surface alloying with nitrogen and carbon. Surf Coat Technol 232:906–911
54. Díaz C, Mandl S, Pereiro R, Fernandez B (2015) Nanomodificated surface Co–Cr alloy for corrosion protection of MoM prosthesis. J Biomater Nanobiotechnol 6(2):91
55. Mani G, Feldman MD, Oh S, Agrawal CM (2009) Surface modification of cobalt–chromium–tungsten–nickel alloy using octadecyltrichlorosilanes. Appl Surf Sci 255(11):5961–5970
56. Bhure R, Mahapatro A, Bonner C, Abdel-Fattah TM (2013) In-vitro stability study of organophosphonic self assembled monolayers (SAMs) on cobalt chromium (Co–Cr) alloy. Mater Sci Eng C 33(4):2050–2058
57. Zhou Z, Wei Q, Li Q, Jiang B, Chen Y, Sun Y (2016) Development of Co-based bulk metallic glasses as potential biomaterials. Mater Sci Eng C 69:46–51
58. Yang ZB, Sun J, Lu S, Vitos L (2018) Assessing elastic property and solid-solution strengthening of binary Ni–Co, Ni–Cr, and ternary Ni–Co–Cr alloys from first-principles theory. J Mater Res 33(18):2763–2774
59. Wang X, Liang Y (2001) Corrosive wear of the Co–Cr–W alloy in liquid zinc. J Mater Res 16(6):1585–1592
60. Sahasrabudhe H, Bose S, Bandyopadhyay A (2018) Laser processed calcium phosphate reinforced CoCrMo for load-bearing applications: processing and wear induced damage evaluation. Acta Biomater 66:118–128
61. Nova K, Novak P, Dvorsky D (2017) Influence of alloying elements on the mechanical properties of a cobalt-based alloy produced with powder metallurgy. Mater Tehnol 51(3):443–447
62. Chiba A, Kumagai K, Nomura N, Miyakawa S (2007) Pin-on-disk wear behavior in a like-on-like configuration in a biological environment of high carbon cast and low carbon forged Co–29Cr–6Mo alloys. Acta Mater 55(4):1309–1318

63. Bose S, Ke D, Sahasrabudhe H, Bandyopadhyay A (2018) Additive manufacturing of biomaterials. Prog Mater Sci 93:45–111
64. Cetiner D, Paksoy AH, Tazegul O, Baydogan M, Guleryuz H, Cimenoglu H, Atar E (2019) A novel fabrication method for a TiO_2 layer over CoCr alloy. Surf Eng 35(3):234–241

Chapter 3
Electrical Discharge Machining for Surface Engineering of Biomedical Alloys

The fabrication of bio-implants using metallic biomaterials presents significant challenges for contemporary manufacturing, particularly when it comes to ensuring long-term clinical functionality. One key difficulty arises from the high hardness and superior wear resistance of standard biomedical alloys, which complicates their machining through conventional techniques. These properties make it challenging to achieve the intricate shapes and fine tolerances that are often required for successful implant integration [1, 2]. Moreover, surface processing is critical, as it greatly influences how well an implant interacts with human tissues and its compatibility within the biological environment. Research conducted by Jenko et al. [3] has demonstrated that machining-induced alterations can significantly impact surface morphology and chemistry, which in turn can enhance cellular responses and promote better healing. For instance, the development of oxide and phosphide layers on the metal surface has been associated with improved bioactivity and increased resistance to intergranular corrosion, both of which are essential for the longevity and safety of implants in the human body. Furthermore, various factors such as tribological behavior, corrosion resistance, and mechanical strength of implants are intrinsically linked to the particular methods utilized for surface treatment. These properties are crucial for ensuring the reliability of implants under physiological conditions, where they are subject to mechanical loads and corrosive biological fluids [4, 5].

Historically, conventional machining techniques have played a vital role in shaping these biomedical components; however, the emergence of non-traditional manufacturing methods has significantly expanded the repertoire available to modern manufacturers. Among these advancements, electrical discharge machining (EDM) stands out as a particularly versatile process. It is capable of creating complex geometries from materials that are otherwise challenging to machine due to their hardness [6, 7]. Research by Lei et al. [8] has illustrated that EDM not only permits precise material removal but also allows for the introduction of advantageous surface characteristics. This can be achieved by incorporating specific powders into the tool electrode or dielectric medium during the machining process, thereby enhancing the

© The Author(s), under exclusive license to Springer Nature Singapore Pte Ltd. 2026

A. Mahajan et al., *Surface Modification of Co–Cr Alloy for Orthopaedic Applications*, Biomedical Materials for Multi-functional Applications,
https://doi.org/10.1007/978-981-95-4029-7_3

functional properties of the implant surfaces. Overall, the continuous development of advanced machining technologies is crucial for overcoming the existing challenges in bio-implant manufacturing, paving the way for innovations that improve patient outcomes and implant longevity.

3.1 Principles of Electro Discharge Machining (EDM)

EDM, or electrical discharge machining, is a manufacturing process that relies on the principle of material removal through controlled electrical discharges. In this technique, a conductive workpiece and a specialized tool, both submerged in a dielectric fluid, engage in a series of rapid electrical discharges. When a voltage is applied between the tool and the workpiece, it establishes a plasma channel, which generates extremely high localized temperatures, typically ranging from 8000 to 10,000 K [9]. These intense electrical sparks result in the melting and vaporization of micro-volumes of material from the workpiece. As the discharges occur, the melted material is effectively flushed away by the dielectric fluid, creating defined craters and leaving behind resolidified zones that reflect the machining process. According to the research conducted by Descoeudres [10], each discharge usually removes an incredibly small volume of material, approximately 10^{-6} to 10^{-4} mm^3. Despite the minuscule size of each removal, the process takes place at a remarkably high frequency, often producing tens of thousands of sparks each second. This rapid succession of discharges leads to significant cumulative material removal over time, allowing for precise and intricate shaping of the workpiece. To help illustrate this process, Fig. 3.1 provides a visual representation of a standard EDM configuration, alongside microstructural images that showcase the fine details of a processed substrate. This comprehensive view highlights both the setup and the results of EDM, underscoring its effectiveness in modern machining applications.

The localized melting and solidification processes associated with electrical discharge machining (EDM) create a distinct modified surface layer on the workpiece. This layer frequently shows significant alterations in both its microstructure and chemical composition, which can influence the overall material properties. During EDM, high-energy discharges generate a plasma that is enriched with ions released from the eroding electrode, as well as ions produced from the decomposition of the dielectric fluid. These characteristics of the plasma contribute to intricate interactions at the material surface, leading to thermal and mechanical effects that modify the microstructure. Consequently, various machining parameters, including pulse duration, polarity, discharge current, and the specific type of dielectric fluid used, play a crucial role in determining the extent and nature of these surface modifications. For instance, adjusting the pulse duration can influence the energy input per discharge, subsequently affecting the depth and quality of the modified layer [11]. Understanding and optimizing these parameters are vital for achieving desired surface characteristics such as hardness, wear resistance, and overall performance of the machined component.

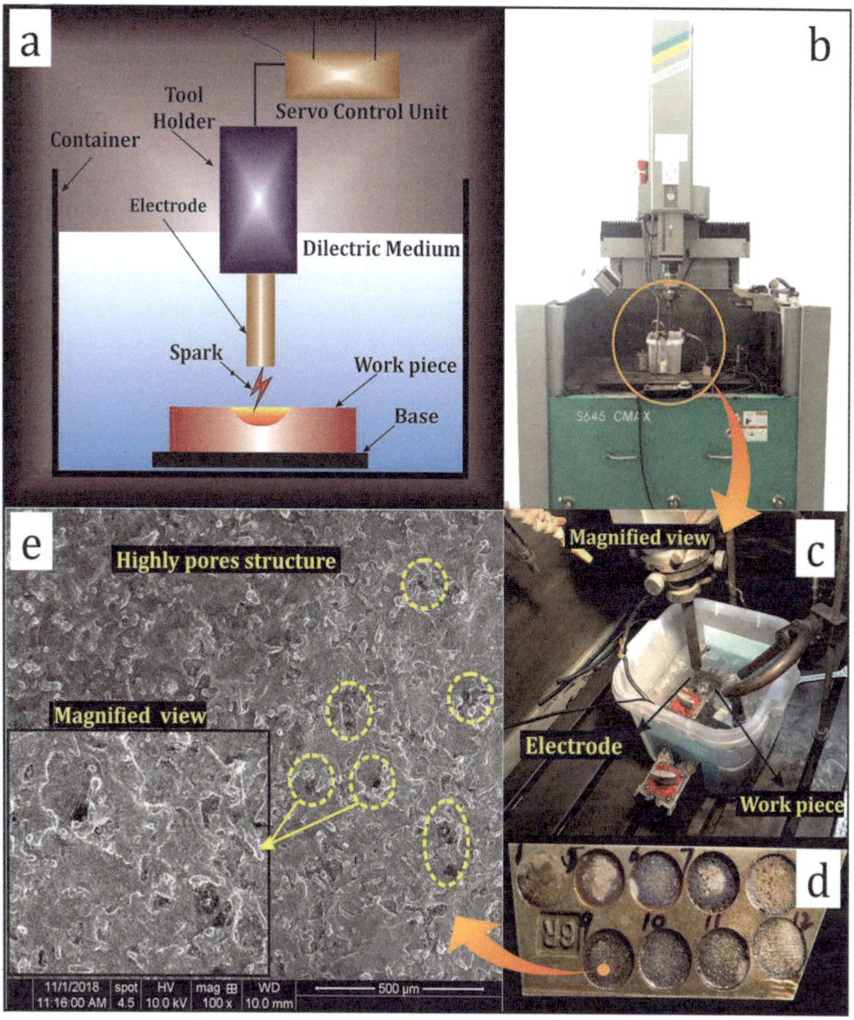

Fig. 3.1 **a** Schematic presentation of EDM setup; **b**, **c** pictographic and magnified view of EDM experimentation; **d** impression on workpiece after machining; **e** scanning electron microscopy image of ED machined substrate. Reproduced with permission from IOP Science [11]

3.2 Background of EDM

The origins of electrical discharge machining (EDM) can be traced back to 1770, when the English scientist Joseph Priestley first observed the erosive potential of electrical discharges. Priestley's pioneering work hinted at the transformative capabilities of electricity, although it would take nearly two centuries for these insights to be applied in manufacturing processes [12]. It was not until the 1930s that scientists began to harness these principles for machining hard materials, such as metals and diamonds. Early experiments in EDM relied on uncontrolled arc discharges between the tool and the workpiece. This method resulted in excessive localized heating, leading to imprecise material removal and potential damage to both the tool and the workpiece. Because of these shortcomings, the process was initially referred to as "arc machining," a term that underscored its lack of precision and control [13]. A significant advancement came in 1943 when Russian engineers B. R. and N. I. Lazarenko developed an innovative system that utilized dielectric fluids to enhance the process. By introducing these fluids, they were able to focus the energy of electrical discharges more effectively, thereby increasing the efficiency and accuracy of material removal. This breakthrough was crucial, as it allowed for sparks to be controlled within a dielectric environment, significantly reducing the mechanical contact between the electrode and the workpiece. Their work established the foundational principles of what is now recognized as modern EDM. Their findings demonstrated that controlled electrical sparks could selectively erode materials with minimal thermal impact, opening up new possibilities for precision machining in industries requiring intricate designs and high-quality finishes [14]. This evolution marked a turning point in manufacturing, paving the way for modern techniques that have since become essential in various applications, from aerospace to medical device manufacturing.

By 1950, the introduction of the resistance–capacitance (RC) type power supply marked a significant milestone in electrical discharge machining (EDM) technology. This innovative power supply allowed for improved control over spark timing, which is crucial for the accuracy of the machining process. Additionally, it included automatic adjustments for the gap between the electrode and the workpiece, optimizing performance and efficiency. As a result, this advancement expanded the practical applications of EDM, making it particularly effective for tasks such as the removal of broken taps, common challenges in machining, and precision drilling in hydraulic systems, which require exact dimensions and reliability [15]. The evolution of EDM continued into the 1980s with the integration of computer systems, which revolutionized the machining industry. The advent of computer numerical control (CNC) introduced significant enhancements, allowing for greater accuracy in the machining process and facilitating a new level of process automation [16]. Operators could program complex machining tasks, resulting in improved efficiency and consistency, reducing the chances of human error. The 1990s brought another notable development with the introduction of powder-mixed EDM (PMEDM). In this process, fine powder particles were suspended in the dielectric fluid used during machining. This innovation contributed to enhanced surface integrity of machined components, reducing tool wear and improving the overall quality of the finished product. PMEDM allowed manufacturers to achieve finer surface finishes and better material properties, which is essential in high-tech industries [17]. These advancements have positioned EDM as a highly compelling technology for high-precision applications, particularly in the biomedical sector. Here, the demands for exceptional surface quality and biofunctionality are critical, as they directly impact the performance and safety of medical

Evolution Period	Year	Description	
Beginning Era (1940-1980s)	1770	Evolution of EDM	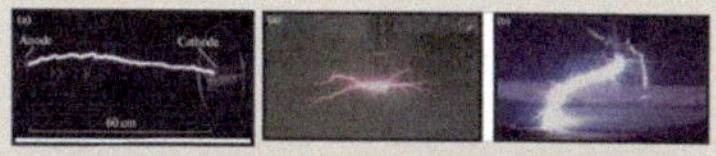
	1930	Innovation of material erosion process in EDM	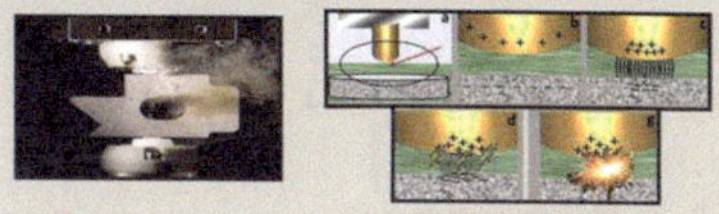
	1950	RC (resistance-capacitance) used as power supply unit in EDM	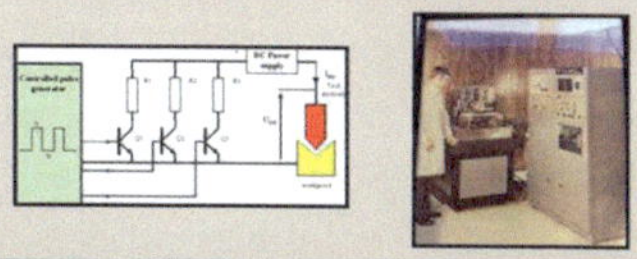
	1980	Computer assisted EDM	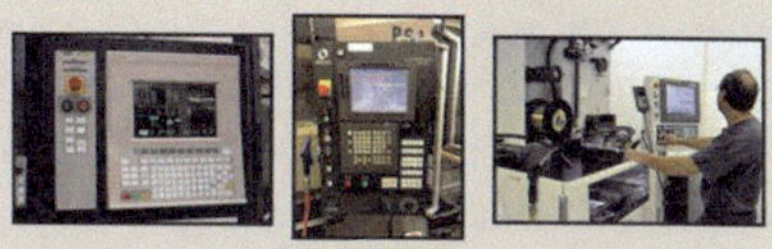
Developing Era (1980s-2000s)	1990	Hybridization of EDM like PMEDM process	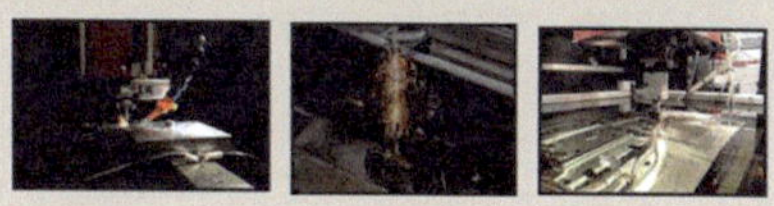
Modren Era (21st century Materials)	2000	EDM in medical field Surface modification by EDM	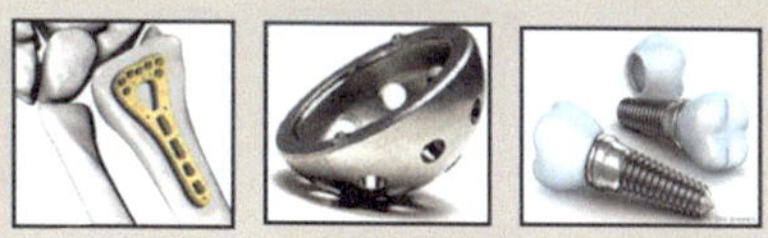

Fig. 3.2 Growth in the EDM process

devices and implants [18–20]. The trajectory of EDM technology is visually represented in Fig. 3.2, highlighting its evolution and the ongoing improvements that continue to shape its applications today.

3.3 Surface Engineering by EDM

Biomedical implants frequently face performance limitations due to ongoing clinical challenges, including chronic inflammation, bacterial colonization, material wear, and corrosion. These issues not only compromise the functionality of the implants but often lead to the necessity for revision surgeries, which can increase healthcare costs and patient morbidity. To tackle these persistent problems, a combination of mechanical and surface treatments is employed to improve the interaction between implants, surrounding tissues, and bone structures. Surface engineering is a critical element in this process, as it directly influences the biomechanical integration of the implant. By enhancing uniform stress transfer and increasing biological acceptance, surface modifications can significantly improve the overall performance and longevity of the implant. This engineering process involves altering the surface characteristics, such as roughness, hydrophilicity, and chemical composition, while preserving the core properties of the material. Techniques used in surface engineering may include the removal of existing surface layers through methods such as abrasive blasting or polishing, as well as the deposition of functional coatings that impart specific chemical and physical properties to the surface. From a clinical perspective, these surface modifications are essential for facilitating bone regeneration and promoting optimal healing conditions. Engineered surfaces can dramatically influence crucial biological processes, including cell adhesion, protein absorption, and the host body's overall biological response. For example, a roughened surface can improve osteointegration by allowing for better attachment of bone-forming cells. Similarly, hydrophilic coatings can enhance wettability, which aids in protein adsorption essential for healing.

Among various surface engineering techniques, electrical discharge machining (EDM) stands out due to its unique ability to precisely shape material while also modifying surface chemistry. EDM not only allows for intricate designs that can enhance mechanical interlocks between the implant and bone but it also enables control over surface characteristics that can encourage favorable biological responses. This dual capability makes EDM a powerful tool in the development of advanced biomedical implants that can better withstand the challenges presented in clinical settings. Such innovations hold the potential to extend the lifespan of implants and reduce the need for subsequent surgeries, ultimately improving patient outcomes and quality of life.

3.3.1 Influence of EDM Parameters on Surface Modification

The effectiveness of surface modification using EDM is intricately linked to the precise tuning of several critical process parameters [21]. Key variables, including discharge current, pulse duration, off-time (pause), voltage, polarity, tool material, and the type of dielectric fluid, all play a significant role in determining both the characteristics of the surface produced and the rate of material removal [22, 23]. Among these parameters, discharge current, typically measured in amperes, emerges as the most pivotal factor. The discharge current dictates the energy delivered during each electrical discharge, which directly influences the resulting surface texture of the machined material. Higher current levels result in more aggressive material erosion, leading to distinct surface features such as pronounced cavities and rough textures. Conversely, lower current settings yield smoother finishes, suitable for applications requiring fine surface qualities. For instance, experiments with machining titanium alloy (Ti–6Al–4V) using graphite electrodes at current levels ranging from 21 to 79 A have demonstrated that higher currents tend to create coarser surfaces that are enriched with carbon. This unique surface characteristic may significantly enhance the alloy's biological performance through increased surface roughness, which can improve cell adhesion and growth. Another critical parameter is pulse duration, often referred to as on-time [24]. Longer pulse durations result in the generation of deeper and wider craters, as a greater amount of energy is imparted with each discharge. This phenomenon has been documented in studies conducted by Kumar et al. [25] and Singh et al. [26], which report a general increase in material removal rates with longer pulse times. However, this also tends to create a rougher surface finish, which may not be desirable in all applications. On the other hand, the pulse interval, or pause time, plays a vital role in stabilizing the electrical discharge and facilitating the effective evacuation of debris produced during the machining process. A well-optimized pulse interval ensures that molten particles are adequately flushed away, thus minimizing the formation of recast layers and reducing the risk of arcing, which can compromise both surface quality and tool life [27]. Moreover, the concept of duty factor, which relates to pulse duration, cannot be overlooked. The duty cycle is defined as the ratio of the pulse duration to the total cycle time, illustrating the proportion of time the spark is actively engaged in material removal (Fig. 3.3a). This parameter is essential for balancing productivity with the desired surface quality, as it influences both the efficiency of the machining process and the final characteristics of the workpiece surface. Overall, a comprehensive understanding of these parameters and their interplay is crucial for optimizing the EDM process, ensuring that the desired surface modifications are achieved while maintaining efficiency and tool longevity. It is expressed as:

$$\text{Duty Factor (\%)} = \frac{\text{Pulse Duration (On-Time) } (\mu\text{s})}{\text{Total Cycle Time (On-Time + Pause Time) } (\mu\text{s})} * 100 \quad (3.1)$$

Discharge voltage is a critical parameter in EDM, as it significantly influences the machining process. Higher open-circuit voltages increase the width of the spark gap, which directly enhances the flushing mechanism. This improved flushing allows for better removal of debris and byproducts, resulting in superior machining efficiency and surface finish [28]. However, it's important to note that while the discharge voltage can greatly improve surface quality, its impact on the overall surface hardness of the workpiece is typically minimal. The selection of electrode materials is another vital aspect of the EDM process [29, 30]. Commonly used materials include copper, graphite, brass, and tungsten. Each of these materials must demonstrate excellent electrical conductivity and resistance to arcing to ensure effective operation. The type of electrode not only influences the rate of tool wear but also plays a significant role in determining the final surface chemistry and morphology of the workpiece being machined [31]. For instance, some materials may impart different elemental compositions or alter the surface texture, which can affect the performance of the final product. Polarity in EDM defines the direction of current flow during the discharge process. In a straight polarity setup, the electrode (tool) acts as the cathode, while the workpiece is the anode [32, 33]. Conversely, in reverse polarity, these roles are switched. Notably, reverse polarity often leads to an increased transfer

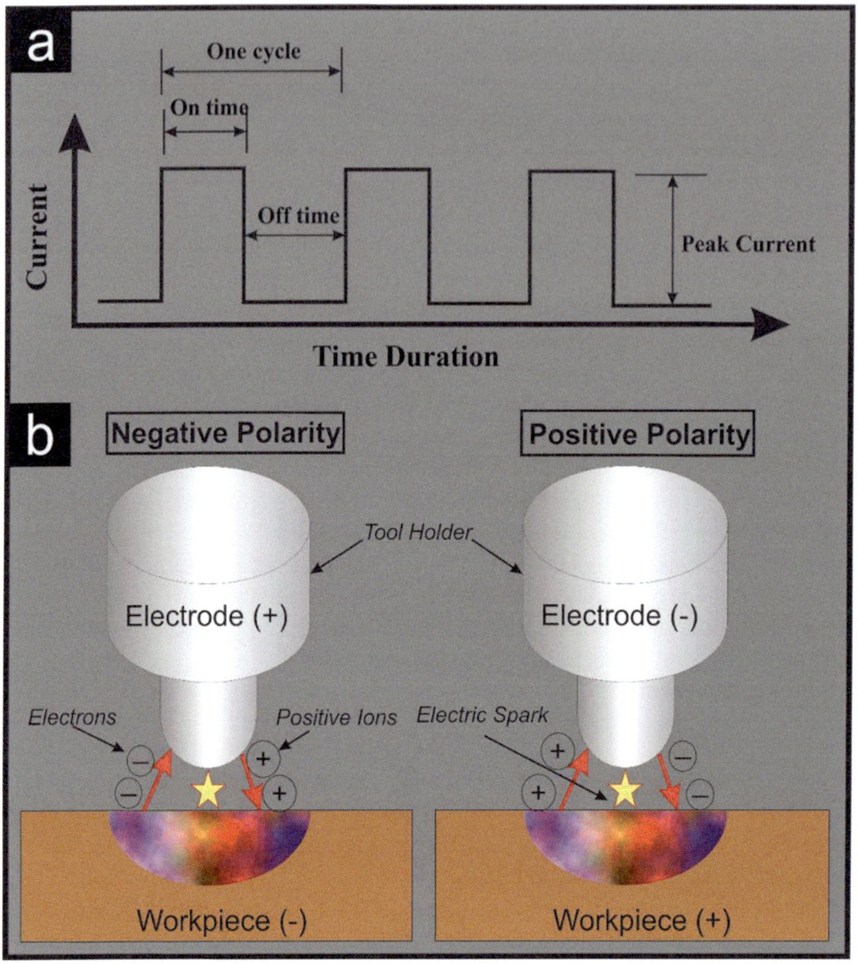

Fig. 3.3 **a** Pulse wavelength; **b** polarity setting in EDM

of electrode material to the workpiece, which can create a hardened surface layer that alters the microstructure of the material. Research indicates that while reverse polarity enhances the material removal rate and increases tool wear, it also results in a finished product that may have different properties compared to that produced with straight polarity [34]. In contrast, straight polarity generally improves surface hardness, making it a preferred choice for applications where hardness is critical. To illustrate, Fig. 3.3b depicts the polarity settings utilized in the EDM process, visually representing the differences and applications of straight versus reverse polarity. Understanding these dynamics is essential for optimizing machining operations and tailoring results to meet specific engineering requirements.

The dielectric fluid is essential in EDM and serves several critical functions. Firstly, it regulates the spark gap, ensuring that the electrical discharge occurs at the optimal distance between the electrode and the workpiece. Secondly, the fluid provides insulation until the dielectric strength is exceeded, preventing unintended discharges that could lead to machining errors. Additionally, it effectively flushes away debris generated during the machining process, which helps maintain a clear working area and enhances tool performance. There are various types of dielectric media available, including hydrocarbon oils and deionized water, each offering unique benefits. Hydrocarbon oils, for instance, are known for their excellent cooling properties and high flash points, making them suitable for high-energy applications. In contrast, deionized water typically has a lower viscosity and can provide better flushing efficiency, particularly for fine machining operations. The proper selection and management of the dielectric fluid are vital for optimizing machining efficiency and ensuring surface integrity. Studies have demonstrated that the right choice of fluid can lead to improved material removal rates, reduced electrode wear, and better surface finishes. Understanding the properties of different dielectric fluids and how they interact with the machining environment can significantly impact the overall success of EDM processes, as highlighted in various research studies [35, 36].

3.4 Biomedical Applications of Conventional EDM-Treated Surfaces

Traditional electrical discharge machining (EDM) processes have proven to be highly effective in enhancing the surface performance of biomedical alloys, making them increasingly relevant in the field of medical implants. Numerous studies have validated the capability of EDM to impart favorable tribological (friction and wear) and biological properties to the surfaces of alloys used in various implant applications. For instance, in a notable study by Philip et al. [37], the researchers employed EDM on the Ti–6Al–4V alloy, a common material used for orthopedic implants, to evaluate its changes in wear resistance and friction behavior. Their results demonstrated that the EDM process facilitated the formation of protective oxide and carbide films on the alloy's surface, which significantly enhanced its wear performance. These findings underline the potential of EDM to prolong the lifespan of implants by reducing wear-related failures. In a different approach, Chen et al. [38] explored a hybrid machining setup that integrated EDM with ultrasonic vibrations to treat an Al–Zn–Mg alloy, frequently used in biomedical applications due to its favorable strength-to-weight ratio. The hybrid method resulted in superior surface quality and the development of a dense surface layer compared to traditional EDM techniques. This advancement demonstrates the potential for combining different machining methods to optimize surface characteristics further, ultimately leading to better implant performance. EDM has thus emerged as a promising surface modification technique, capable of significantly enhancing the biofunctionality of metallic implants. It produces surfaces that not only exhibit improved adhesion and mechanical interlocking but also enhance corrosion resistance, factors that are critical for the long-term success of implants in-vivo. For example, in the study conducted by Harcuba et al. [24], the researchers focused on EDM-treated Ti–6Al–4V alloy and reported exceptionally high cellular compatibility when compared to substrates that were coated with TiO_2 using traditional techniques. The improved interaction of cells with the EDM-treated surfaces can be attributed to the presence of microscale surface irregularities, which promote better cell anchorage and proliferation. Additionally, the stable carbon-enriched recast layer formed during the EDM process further supports osteoblast proliferation, an essential aspect for successful bone integration. Overall, these insights emphasize the significant potential of EDM not only to enhance the mechanical properties of biomedical alloys but also to promote their biological performance, paving the way for the development of more effective and durable implants in the medical field.

Yang et al. [39] reported significant advancements in the machining of titanium alloys using electrical discharge machining at high current levels. This technique led to the formation of nanostructured oxide layers on the titanium surfaces, which notably enhanced cell adhesion and increased biological activity, making these surfaces more conducive to integration with biological tissues. In a related study, Lee et al. [40] noted that osteoblasts, the cells responsible for bone formation, exhibited improved responses when cultured on Ti6Al4V surfaces treated through EDM, suggesting that the process fosters an environment favorable for bone integration. Murali et al. [41] employed a micro-EDM approach to fabricate bioactive surfaces on Ti6Al4V implants. They incorporated ultrasonic vibration during the machining process, which played a vital role in reducing surface roughness. The cavitation effect generated by the ultrasound not only helped to remove debris efficiently but also resulted in smoother surfaces that remained within the clinically acceptable roughness threshold of 0.4 μm. This refinement in surface quality is crucial for enhancing biocompatibility, as smoother surfaces are more likely to support cell adhesion and proliferation.

Research led by Mahmud et al. [42] focused on utilizing EDM with pulse power control to create micro-pits on artificial hip implants. The primary aim of this micropitting was to improve lubrication, thereby reducing wear and extending the lifespan of the implants. In another notable study, Klocke et al. [43] innovatively combined EDM with plasma electrolytic conversion for the surface modification of magnesium implants. This hybrid technique was effective in enhancing both the corrosion resistance and bioactivity of the biodegradable magnesium material, addressing the challenges often faced with traditional implants that can lead to adverse biological responses over time. EDM has also emerged as a clinically relevant technique in the field of dentistry, particularly for the production of passive-fitting implants that ensure better structural integrity and patient comfort. Zinelis et al. [44] evaluated the effects of EDM on dental alloys and discovered a substantial increase in hardness attributable to the formation of a protective oxide layer. They also reported improved fit between prosthetic superstructures and abutments, which contributes to more efficient stress transfer and enhanced mechanical stability in dental applications. Additionally, Bhui et al. [45] revealed that surfaces treated with EDM showed not only improved biological responses but also increased wear resistance. This was linked to the formation of intermetallics, silicides, and carbides during the EDM process. These modifications resulted in surfaces with superior corrosion resistance, reinforcing EDM's potential for use in orthopedic applications where long-term durability is paramount. Furthermore, Shin et al. [46] highlighted the advantages of creating porous surfaces via EDM, noting that these porous structures significantly promote tissue integration. The increased surface area and interconnectivity of pores facilitate cellular in-growth, which is essential for successful implant integration in biological systems. Overall, the diverse applications and benefits of EDM underscore its importance in both orthopedic and dental fields, making it a vital technology for the advancement of implant materials and their performance in clinical settings.

Peng et al. [47] conducted EDM utilizing copper electrodes and distilled water to develop advanced nanostructured titanium surfaces. Their innovative approach involved short spark durations accompanied by hydrogen generation, which collectively contributed to the formation of highly bioactive textures on the titanium surface. This bioactivity is essential for applications in biomedical fields where enhanced interaction with biological tissues is desired. Chang-Bin et al. [48] explored the effects of EDM on titanium alloys, revealing that EDM-based coatings significantly improved both the tribological (friction and wear) and mechanical properties of these alloys. Furthermore, their research emphasized a notable enhancement in the biological behavior of titanium, making it more suitable for medical implants and other biological applications. Mahajan et al. [49] built upon these findings by investigating the effects of EDM on cobalt-chromium (Co–Cr) alloys. Their studies demonstrated that EDM-treated Co–Cr specimens exhibited superior corrosion resistance and biocompatibility when compared to untreated samples. This improvement was particularly noteworthy, as it was shown to enhance MG-63 cell adhesion and promote red blood cell formation, both critical factors for the use of these materials in biological environments. Following this research, they expanded their research to include duplex stainless steel (DSS-2205), applying the same EDM technique [50, 51]. Their findings indicated an impressive increase of up to 90% in both corrosion resistance and biological response in the treated samples. They attributed these substantial benefits to the formation of protective carbide and oxide layers, which arose from the interactions between the alloy and the dielectric fluid used during the EDM process. These layers not only protect the underlying material from corrosive environments but also enhance its overall durability.

In another study, Ablyaz et al. [52] examined the wear characteristics of EDM-treated duplex stainless steel (DSS) alloys. Their results revealed fewer cracks and significantly enhanced wear resistance compared to unmachined samples, indicating that the EDM process had a clear positive impact on the structural integrity of the material. Figure 3.4 illustrates the wear characteristics through FE-SEM images, showcasing the differences between untreated and EDM-machined surfaces. Specifically, the ED-machined surface displayed minimal cracking and no signs of delamination, underscoring its exceptional wear resistance compared to the unmachined alloy specimens. This research collectively highlights the transformative potential of

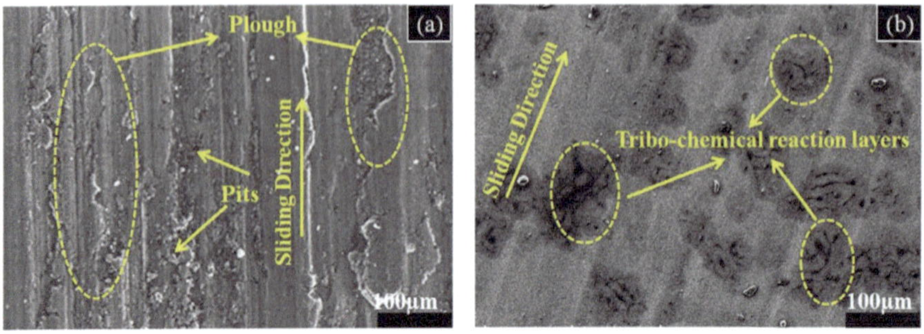

Fig. 3.4 Wear images of **a** unmachined specimen; **b** ED machined specimen. Reproduced under license CC-BY-4.0 [52]

EDM treatments in enhancing the properties of various alloy materials for advanced applications.

3.5 Applications of Powder-Mixed EDM in Biomedical Surface Engineering

Recent advancements have positioned powder-mixed electrical discharge machining (PMEDM) as an innovative and leading technique for the modification of biomedical surfaces, particularly in the context of enhancing the longevity and functionality of metal implants. This technique involves the dispersion of electrically conductive powders, such as silicon carbide, titanium, or other specialized materials, into the dielectric fluid used during the machining process. By doing so, PMEDM alters the breakdown strength of the fluid and expands the spark gap between the electrode and the workpiece. This crucial adjustment allows for more efficient energy distribution during the machining process, resulting in improved machining efficiency and superior surface characteristics [53]. Research by Xu et al. [54] has highlighted PMEDM's potential in the deposition of functional surface coatings, which significantly enhance both the mechanical strength and biological performance of metal implants. These coatings can lead to improvements in wear resistance and fatigue strength, which are vital for implants subjected to mechanical stress within the body. In another study, Huang et al. [55] discovered that surfaces treated with PMEDM exhibited not only enhanced corrosion resistance, crucial for implants exposed to bodily fluids, but also improved wear durability and biocompatibility, making them more suitable for long-term use within biological environments. Li et al. [56] took the investigation further by integrating silicon carbide (SiC) powder into the dielectric fluid during the machining of titanium alloys. They observed the formation of a thick, uniform recast layer on the titanium surface. This recast layer is instrumental in enhancing surface integrity, as it can improve the mechanical interlocking of the implant with surrounding bone tissue, thereby facilitating better integration and stability within the body. In a complementary study, Chen et al. [57] employed titanium powder in deionized water during the PMEDM process to fabricate a hydrophilic, crack-free layer on titanium implants. The hydrophilic nature of this layer proves beneficial for osseointegration, as it can promote the attachment and proliferation of osteoblasts, the cells responsible for bone formation. This tailored approach to surface engineering underscores the versatility and effectiveness of PMEDM in advancing biomedical applications, ultimately contributing to improved patient outcomes and the success of implant procedures.

Silver powder has garnered significant attention in recent years due to its notable antimicrobial properties. Research conducted by Bui et al. [58] demonstrated that the incorporation of silver into dielectric fluid markedly improved the antibacterial characteristics of titanium surfaces. This enhancement is crucial for biomedical applications, where the prevention of bacterial infections is paramount. In another study, Sales et al. [59] utilized calcium chloride ($CaCl_2$) within the dielectric to facilitate the deposition of a calcium-rich coating on Ti6Al4V substrates. This innovative process not only resulted in the formation of calcium titanate ($CaTiO_3$) but also produced various surface features, such as pits and globules, which can enhance cell attachment and biological functionality in implant applications. The application of PMEDM has been explored as a cost-effective method for generating oxide layers on titanium alloys. This technique allows for precise engineering of surfaces, making them suitable for medical implants. Notably, the incorporation of hydroxyapatite (HAp) powder into the dielectric has proven effective in forming bioactive TiO_2-based coatings, which are crucial for promoting bone integration [60]. Furthermore, Sharma et al. [61] investigated the use of zirconium and manganese powders in conjunction with a biodegradable Mg–4Zn alloy, achieving a remarkable reduction in corrosion rates of over 40% when compared to untreated samples. This significant improvement not only enhances the longevity of the alloy in physiological environments but also minimizes risks associated with corrosion-related failures. In another study, Razak et al. [62] focused on the use of zinc powder in the dielectric during the machining of magnesium alloys. Their findings indicated that this approach resulted in surfaces with reduced roughness and lower corrosion rates. The observed effects are attributed to consistent energy dispersion during the sparking process, which leads to improved surface integrity. Prakash et al. [63] conducted a comparative analysis of untreated, EDM-treated, and PMEDM-treated titanium alloys in the context of their interaction with MG-63 osteoblast cells, a type of bone cell. The results revealed that PMEDM-modified surfaces significantly enhanced cell adhesion and proliferation, indicating a superior level of biocompatibility essential for successful implant integration. The cellular interactions were visually documented through scanning electron microscopy (SEM), with the detailed images provided in Fig. 3.5. This comprehensive understanding of surface modifications underscores the potential for advanced materials in biomedical applications.

Sadat-Shojai et al. [64] emphasized the critical role of hydroxyapatite (HAp) coatings in enhancing implant-tissue integration. These coatings effectively reduce ion release from implants, which is crucial for maintaining a stable biological environment and promoting positive cellular responses. Öpöz et al. [65] conducted

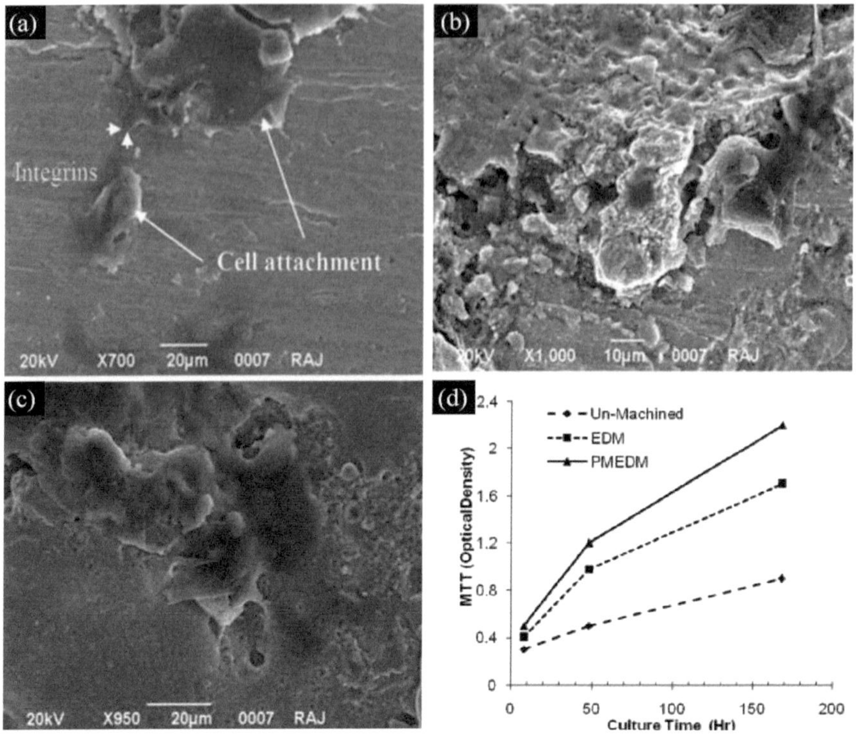

Fig. 3.5 MG-63 cell attachment on **a** untreated substrate; **b** ED machined substrate; **c** PMED machined substrate; **d** MTT assay of MG63 cells after culture for 1, 3 and 7 days. Reproduced with permission from Elsevier [63]

experiments that demonstrated that incorporating HAp into deionized water during the PMEDM process created smooth and bioactive surfaces that lacked significant cracks, which are often detrimental to the integration process. Further supporting this research, Singh et al. [66] and Yaşar et al. [67] reported that titanium surfaces treated with HAp exhibited improved corrosion resistance and wear performance. This enhancement not only extends the lifespan of the implants but also promotes better compatibility with surrounding cells, crucial for successful integration into the body. Additionally, Lamichhane et al. [68] evaluated the influence of HAp coatings on 316L stainless steel, a commonly used material in medical implants. Their findings indicated substantial improvements in biocompatibility, suggesting that HAp coatings can significantly enhance the interaction between the implant and biological tissues. The differences in surface characteristics are illustrated in SEM imaging presented in Fig. 3.6. This figure contrasts the coarse and damaged surfaces typically found on conventionally machined substrates with the smoother and more porous textures achieved through PMEDM when using HAp powder. These findings collectively indicate that HAp coatings not only improve the mechanical properties of

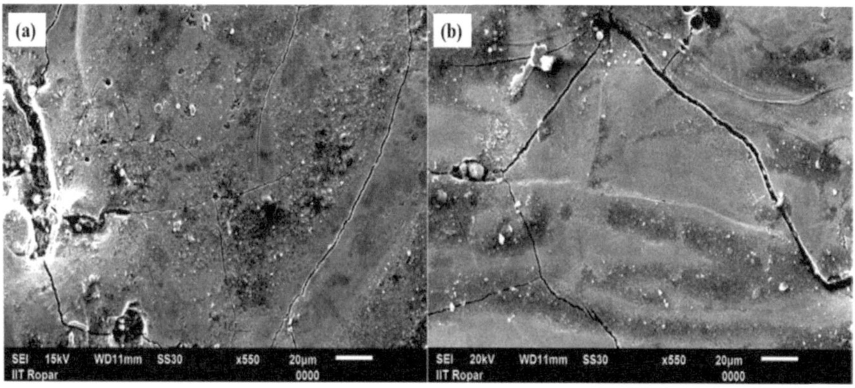

Fig. 3.6 SEM images of **a** conventional ED machined substrate; **b** PMED machined substrate. Reproduced with permission from Elsevier [68]

implants but also foster a more biocompatible environment conducive to successful tissue integration.

Carbon nanotubes (CNTs) have gained considerable attention in the field of PMEDM due to their exceptional mechanical and electrical properties. These nanomaterials exhibit remarkable strength-to-weight ratios and high electrical conductivity, which enhance their functionality in machining applications [69]. During the PMEDM process, CNTs are uniformly dispersed within the dielectric fluid, which optimizes thermal conduction and significantly reduces the formation of surface defects on the machined components. Research by Li et al. [70] demonstrated that coating materials with CNTs leads to notable improvements in microhardness, wear resistance, and bioactivity. These enhancements make CNT-coated materials particularly suitable for use in load-bearing biomedical devices, such as implants and prosthetics, where mechanical integrity and biological compatibility are crucial. In a different study, Al-Amin et al. [71] explored a hybrid dielectric system that combines hydroxyapatite (HAp), a material known for its biocompatibility and osteoconductive properties, with CNTs for machining 316L stainless steel. Their findings showed that this innovative approach resulted in significantly increased material removal rates and superior surface finish, indicating a promising direction for enhancing the performance of surgical tools and implants. Devgan et al. [72] further extended the applicability of CNTs by employing multi-walled carbon nanotubes (MWCNTs) in PMEDM for treating beta-type titanium alloys, which are often used in the aerospace and medical industries. Their investigation revealed that the addition of MWCNTs facilitates the formation of a dense and well-bonded remelted layer on the titanium surface. This enhanced layer is critical for improving the material's fatigue strength and corrosion resistance. Notably, as illustrated in Fig. 3.7a, b, the MWCNT-coated surfaces demonstrated strong adhesive properties, with no delamination observed even after undergoing rigorous mechanical testing, as depicted in Fig. 3.7c [73]. Overall, Table 3.1 provides a comprehensive summary of various studies that compare conventional electro-discharge machining (EDM) and PMEDM techniques, highlighting their effectiveness in enhancing the surface properties of different biomedical alloys. This comparative analysis underscores the potential of CNTs and hybrid dielectric systems in advancing the technology and application of precision machining in the biomedical field.

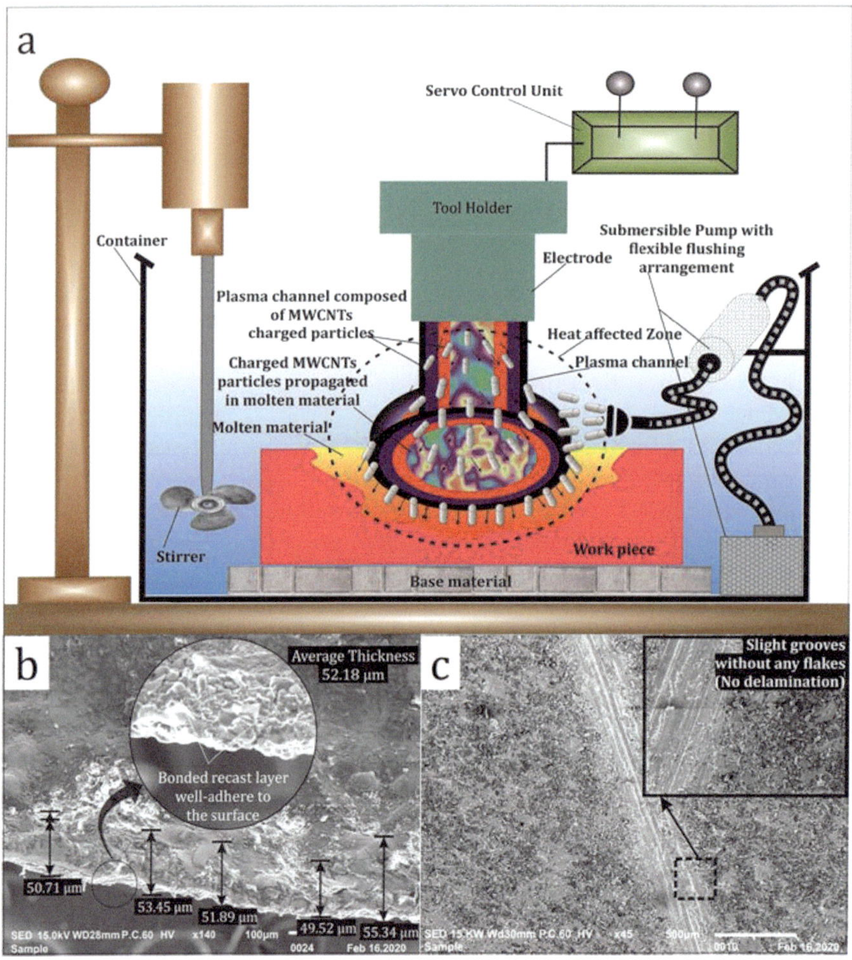

Fig. 3.7 **a** Schematic view of MWCNTs mixed EDM; **b**, **c** FE-SEM images of MWCNTs treated substrate; **b** cross-sectional morphology, **c** adhesion obtained after a 2 mm scratch length. Reproduced with permission from Springer Nature [73]

Table 3.1 Summary of the literature using EDM technique for surface alteration of different alloys

Process	Alloy	Properties improved after surface modification by electric discharge machining					Material removal rate	References
		Corrosion resistance	Tribological characteristics	Biocompatibility	Surface quality	Micro-hardness		
EDM	Ti6Al4V	–	✓	–	–	–	–	[37]
		–	–	✓	–	–	–	[24]
		–	–	✓	–	–	–	[39]
		–	–	✓	–	–	–	[40]
		–	–	✓	✓	–	–	[41]
		–	–	–	✓	✓	–	[44]
		✓	✓	✓	–	–	–	[45]
		✓	✓	✓	–	–	–	[48]
	Co–Cr–Mo	–	–	–	✓	–	✓	[21]
		✓	✓	✓	✓	–	–	[49]
	F67 grade IV titanium sheet	–	–	✓	–	–	–	[47]
	DSS	✓	–	✓	–	–	–	[50, 51]
		–	✓	–	–	–	–	[52]
EDM with ultrasonic machining	Al–Zn–Mg	–	–	–	✓	✓	–	[38]
EDM with plasma	Magnesium	–	–	✓	–	–	–	[43]
PMEDM	Ti6Al4V	–	–	✓	✓	✓	–	[56]
		–	–	✓	–	–	–	[58]

(continued)

Table 3.1 (continued)

Process	Alloy	Properties improved after surface modification by electric discharge machining					Material removal rate	References
		Corrosion resistance	Tribological characteristics	Biocompatibility	Surface quality	Micro-hardness		
		–	–	✓	✓	✓	–	[59]
		–	–	✓	✓	–	–	[60]
		–	–	✓	✓	–	–	[65]
		✓	✓	–	–	–	–	[66]
		–	–	✓	✓	–	–	[67]
		–	✓	✓	–	✓	–	[70]
	Ti (β-type)	–	–	✓	–	–	–	[63]
		–	✓	✓	–	✓	–	[72, 73]
	Grade 4 pure Ti	–	–	✓	✓	–	–	[57]
	Mg alloy	✓	–	–	–	–	✓	[61]
		✓	–	–	✓	–	–	[51]
	316L SS	–	–	✓	–	–	–	[68]
		–	–	✓	–	–	✓	[71]

3.6 Discussion and Overall Summary

Electrical discharge machining has become a highly effective technique for modifying the surface characteristics of biomedical alloys, marking a significant advancement in the field of medical technology. This method not only enhances biocompatibility, ensuring that the materials are well-received by the body, but also improves corrosion resistance and tribological performance, features crucial for the longevity and effectiveness of medical implants. By manipulating the surface at micro- and nano-levels, EDM promotes better integration with surrounding tissues, which is essential for the success of implants in various medical applications. Despite its advantages, EDM faces specific challenges, particularly when machining hard or tough alloys commonly used in biomedical applications. These materials often exhibit low machinability, which can lead to slower removal rates during the machining process. As a result, higher discharge energies are frequently necessary to achieve the desired depth of material modification. Although employing high-energy discharges can facilitate more profound changes to the material's surface, it also comes with a range of potential drawbacks. For instance, excessive energy can lead to unstable electrical arcs, which may cause microcracks and irregular surface features due to the thermal stresses involved. Such imperfections can significantly diminish the machining quality and ultimately affect the performance of the implant. Moreover, high-energy discharges often create deeper craters and more pronounced surface defects compared to those produced by lower-energy discharges, which can compromise the mechanical properties and biocompatibility of the machined surface. Therefore, it is critical to achieve an optimal balance in the EDM process parameters. This includes careful selection of values for current intensity, pulse duration, and dielectric fluid composition, all of which play a vital role in ensuring effective material removal while maintaining the integrity of the surface. In summary, while EDM offers substantial benefits for enhancing the surface properties of biomedical alloys, careful attention must be paid to the machining conditions to prevent potential negative outcomes, ensuring that the implants meet the rigorous standards required for medical use.

The integration of powders into the dielectric fluid, a fundamental aspect of powder-mixed electrical discharge machining (PMEDM), offers a promising solution for enhancing surface properties in machining processes. This innovative approach not only improves machining efficiency by increasing material removal rates but also enables the production of functionally superior surfaces, which can lead to better performance in various applications. However, several challenges remain to be addressed. For instance, the incorporation of highly conductive powders into the dielectric fluid can disrupt the insulating properties of the dielectric medium. This disruption may result in unstable electrical discharges, which can compromise the quality of the machining process and lead to issues such as excessive cracking or surface degradation in the finished product. Furthermore, while significant advancements have been made in applying EDM and PMEDM techniques to titanium alloys, there is still a notable lack of comprehensive studies examining their effects on other critical materials, such as cobalt-chromium (Co–Cr) alloys and duplex stainless steel (DSS). These materials are often utilized in medical implants and interventional devices due to their excellent biocompatibility and mechanical strength. The current research landscape reveals a gap in experimental data regarding how varying PMEDM parameters, such as pulse duration, powder concentration, and electrode material, affect the biological and mechanical performance of Co–Cr and DSS. Addressing these gaps through targeted research could facilitate wider industrial adoption of PMEDM, particularly in the production of next-generation medical implants that require precise engineering and durability. By exploring diverse combinations of materials and optimizing parameter configurations, future studies could significantly expand the application of EDM and PMEDM in biomedical device manufacturing, ultimately leading to innovations that enhance the performance and longevity of implants while ensuring better patient outcomes.

3.7 Conclusions and Future Scope

Recent studies have provided evidence that surface modification through electrical discharge machining (EDM) can significantly enhance the functional performance of biomedical alloys used in implants. EDM treatments lead to surfaces that exhibit a range of improved biological properties. These include not only increased bioactivity, meaning the surfaces can interact favorably with biological systems, but also enhanced resistance to bacterial adhesion, which is crucial for reducing the risk of infections post-implantation. Additionally, EDM-treated surfaces demonstrate a reduced inflammatory response, contributing to better integration with surrounding tissues. From a mechanical perspective, the advantages of EDM are equally notable. The process contributes to improved corrosion resistance, which is vital for the longevity of implants in the often harsh environments within the human body. Furthermore, EDM can increase surface hardness and wear performance, ensuring that devices remain functional over extended periods. These enhancements are primarily due to the formation of protective surface layers, such as carbides, oxides, and nitrides, during the discharge process. These chemically stable layers not only act as a barrier against degradation but also promote favorable cellular activities, including adhesion and proliferation, which are essential for successful tissue integration. However, it is important to note that the effectiveness of EDM surface treatments hinges on the careful selection of tool materials as well as the precise control of various process parameters. Factors such as discharge energy, pulse duration, and electrode material can greatly influence the quality and characteristics of the treated surface, making the optimization of these variables a critical component of successful EDM implementation in biomedical applications.

Powder-mixed electrical discharge machining (PMEDM) has made significant strides in advancing the capabilities of surface engineering, particularly in the field of biomedical applications. By integrating specialized powders such as carbon nanotubes (CNTs) and nano-hydroxyapatite (μ-HAp) into the dielectric fluid used during the machining process, researchers have successfully improved several key aspects of material performance. These enhancements include increased biocompatibility, superior surface microstructure, and enhanced mechanical properties. The incorporation of these innovative powders not only improves the surface texture of implants but also boosts cellular interactions, which are crucial for promoting tissue integration. Furthermore, the unique properties of CNTs and μ-HAp allow for the creation of surfaces that closely resemble the natural architecture of bone. This resemblance is particularly advantageous for orthopedic and dental applications, where the compatibility of implants with surrounding biological tissues is essential for successful outcomes. Looking to the future, a strong emphasis on multidisciplinary collaboration is vital. Medical researchers, materials scientists, and manufacturing experts must work in tandem to fully exploit the transformative potential of EDM and PMEDM technologies in biomedical engineering. By addressing the existing technological barriers that currently hinder access to advanced bio-implant production, significant progress can be made. Innovative approaches to EDM and PMEDM processes can pave the way for scalable, precise, and cost-effective manufacturing of high-performance implants. Such advancements not only hold promise for improving the quality of medical devices but also have the potential to enhance patient outcomes, making these methods an invaluable part of the future of healthcare technology.

This chapter offers an in-depth analysis for researchers focused on optimizing EDM parameters and selecting appropriate powder combinations. The goal is to engineer advanced surfaces that are specifically designed to enhance osseointegration, the process by which bone integrates with implant surfaces, as well as to extend the longevity of these implants in clinical settings. By examining various EDM techniques and the properties of different powders, this chapter aims to provide valuable insights that can lead to the development of cutting-edge surfaces. Ultimately, these advancements could significantly improve patient outcomes in implant dentistry and orthopedics.

References

1. Philip JT, Mathew J, Kuriachen B (2021) Transition from EDM to PMEDM—impact of suspended particulates in the dielectric on Ti6Al4V and other distinct material surfaces: a review. J Manuf Process 64:1105–1142. https://doi.org/10.1016/J.JMAPRO.2021.01.056
2. Mahajan A, Sidhu SS, Ablyaz T (2019) EDM surface treatment: an enhanced biocompatible interface, pp 33–40. https://doi.org/10.1007/978-981-13-9977-0_3
3. Jenko M, Gorenšek M, Godec M, Hodnik M, Batič BŠ, Donik Č, Grant JT, Dolinar D (2018) Surface chemistry and microstructure of metallic biomaterials for hip and knee endoprostheses. Appl Surf Sci 427:584–593. https://doi.org/10.1016/J.APSUSC.2017.08.007
4. Davis R, Singh A, Jackson MJ, Coelho RT, Prakash D, Charalambous CP, Ahmed W, da Silva LRR, Lawrence AA (2022) A comprehensive review on metallic implant biomaterials and their subtractive manufacturing. Int J Adv Manuf Technol 120(3):1473–1530. https://doi.org/10.1007/S00170-022-08770-8

5. Rahmati M, Silva EA, Reseland JE, Heyward CA, Haugen HJ (2020) Biological responses to physicochemical properties of biomaterial surface. Chem Soc Rev 49:5178–5224. https://doi.org/10.1039/d0cs00103a
6. Mastud S, Garg M, Singh R, Samuel J, Joshi S (2013) Experimental characterization of vibration-assisted reverse micro electrical discharge machining (EDM) for surface texturing. In: ASME 2012 international manufacturing science and engineering conference collocated with the 40th North American manufacturing research conference participation with international conference, MSEC 2012, pp 439–448. https://doi.org/10.1115/MSEC2012-7314
7. Das A, Ambastha S, Priyadarshni N, Samanta S, Nagahanumaiah (2021) Fabrication of hydrophobic surfaces on titanium using micro-EDM exhibiting antibacterial properties. Proc Inst Mech Eng Part B J Eng Manuf 236:1093–1101. https://doi.org/10.1177/09544054211060981
8. Lei J, Wu X, Zhou Z, Xu B, Zhu L, Tang Y (2021) Sustainable mass production of blind multi-microgrooves by EDM with a long-laminated electrode. J Clean Prod 279:123492. https://doi.org/10.1016/J.JCLEPRO.2020.123492
9. Xu M, Li C, Kurniawan R, Chen J, Ko TJ (2022) Influence of different dielectrics on process performance for electrical discharge-assisted milling of titanium alloy. https://doi.org/10.21203/rs.3.rs-1184922/v1
10. Descoeudres A (2006) Characterization of electrical discharge machining plasmas, no 3542, p 137. https://doi.org/10.5075/EPFL-THESIS-3542
11. Mahajan A, Devgan S, Kalyanasundaram D (2022) Electrical discharge machining—a futuristic technique for surface engineering of biomedical alloys: a concise review. Surf Topogr Metrol Prop 10:043001. https://doi.org/10.1088/2051-672X/ACA9E7
12. Almeida ST, Mo J, Bil C, Ding S, Wang X (2021) Conceptual design of a high-speed wire EDM robotic end-effector based on a systematic review followed by TRIZ. Machines 9:132. https://doi.org/10.3390/MACHINES9070132
13. Ho KH, Newman ST (2003) State of the art electrical discharge machining (EDM). Int J Mach Tools Manuf 43:1287–1300. https://doi.org/10.1016/S0890-6955(03)00162-7
14. Majumder H, Maity K (2018) Prediction and optimization of surface roughness and micro-hardness using GRNN and MOORA-fuzzy—a MCDM approach for nitinol in WEDM. Measurement 118:1–13. https://doi.org/10.1016/J.MEASUREMENT.2018.01.003
15. Abdullah MA, Yahya A, Shukri WN (2020)Integrated control of electrical discharge machining (EDM) using PSoC. J Phys Conf Ser 1529:042087. https://doi.org/10.1088/1742-6596/1529/4/042087
16. Kumar S, Singh R, Singh TP, Sethi BL (2009) Surface modification by electrical discharge machining: a review. J Mater Process Technol 209:3675–3687. https://doi.org/10.1016/J.JMATPROTEC.2008.09.032
17. Kansal HK, Singh S, Kumar P (2007) Technology and research developments in powder mixed electric discharge machining (PMEDM). J Mater Process Technol 184:32–41. https://doi.org/10.1016/J.JMATPROTEC.2006.10.046
18. Uno Y, Okada A, Yamada T, Hayashi Y, Tabuchi Y (1998) Surface integrity in EDM of aluminum bronze with nickel powder mixed fluid. J Japan Soc Electr Mach Eng 32:24–31. https://doi.org/10.2526/JSEME.32.70_24
19. Arantes LJ, da Silva ER, dos Santos RF, Sales WF, Raslan AA (2016) The electrical discharge machining process aided by abrasive jet. Int J Adv Manuf Technol 87(1):411–420. https://doi.org/10.1007/S00170-016-8517-4
20. Perumal A, Kailasanathan C, Stalin B, Rajkumar PR, Gangadharan T, Venkatesan G (2021) Evaluation of EDM process parameters on titanium alloy through Taguchi approach. Mater Today Proc 45:2394–2400. https://doi.org/10.1016/J.MATPR.2020.10.737
21. Yavari R, Esmaeilzadeh A, Razavykia A, Yavari MR, Iranmanesh S (2016) Effect of electrode material and electrical discharge machining parameters on machining of Co–Cr–Mo. Int J Mech Mechatron Eng IJMME-IJENS 16. https://www.researchgate.net/publication/303785239. Accessed 15 Nov 2021

22. Mahajan A, Devgan S, Kalyanasundaram D (2022) Surface alteration of cobalt-chromium and duplex stainless steel alloys for biomedical applications: a concise review. https://doi.org/10.1080/10426914.2022.2105873
23. Prakash C, Kansal HK, Pabla BS, Puri S (2016) Experimental investigations in powder mixed electric discharge machining of Ti–35Nb–7Ta–5Zrβ-titanium alloy. Mater Manuf Process 32:274–285. https://doi.org/10.1080/10426914.2016.1198018
24. Harcuba P, Bačáková L, Stráský J, Bačáková M, Novotná K, Janeček M (2012) Surface treatment by electric discharge machining of Ti–6Al–4V alloy for potential application in orthopaedics. J Mech Behav Biomed Mater 7:96–105. https://doi.org/10.1016/J.JMBBM.2011.07.001
25. Kumar S, Dhingra AK, Kumar S (2017) Parametric optimization of powder mixed electrical discharge machining for nickel-based superalloy inconel-800 using response surface methodology. Mech Adv Mater Mod Process 3(1):1–17. https://doi.org/10.1186/S40759-017-0022-4
26. Kansal HK, Singh S, Kumar P (2005) Parametric optimization of powder mixed electrical discharge machining by response surface methodology. J Mater Process Technol 169:427–436. https://doi.org/10.1016/J.JMATPROTEC.2005.03.028
27. Sisodiya MS, Shukla S, Bajpai V (2022) Feasibility analysis of novel Maglev EDM by comparing with conventional micro EDM. Sci Rep 12(1):1–13. https://doi.org/10.1038/s41598-022-06662-1
28. Kansal HK, Singh S, Kumar P (2005) Application of Taguchi method for optimisation of powder mixed electrical discharge machining. Int J Manuf Technol Manag 7:329–341. https://doi.org/10.1504/IJMTM.2005.006836
29. Rizwee M, Rao PS, Khan MY (2021) Recent advancement in electric discharge machining of metal matrix composite materials. Mater Today Proc 37:2829–2836. https://doi.org/10.1016/J.MATPR.2020.08.657
30. Vidya S, Wattal R, Rao PV (2022) Experimental investigation on machinability and geometric tolerance in die-sinking EDM of microholes and channels. MAPAN 37(2):399–407. https://doi.org/10.1007/S12647-022-00532-X
31. Mahajan A, Sidhu SS, Devgan S (2020) MRR and surface morphological analysis of electrical-discharge-machined Co–Cr alloy. Emerg Mater Res 9:42–46. https://doi.org/10.1680/JEMMR.19.00034
32. Muthuramalingam T, Mohan B, Jothilingam A (2014) Effect of tool electrode resolidification on surface hardness in electrical discharge machining. Mater Manuf Process 29:1374–1380. https://doi.org/10.1080/10426914.2014.930956
33. Mughal MP, Farooq MU, Mumtaz J, Mia M, Shareef M, Javed M, Jamil M, Pruncu CI (2021) Surface modification for osseointegration of Ti6Al4V ELI using powder mixed sinking EDM. J Mech Behav Biomed Mater 113:104145. https://doi.org/10.1016/J.JMBBM.2020.104145
34. Kumar S, Singh R, Batish A, Singh TP (2016) Investigations on effect of electrode polarity on machining performance of Ti-5Al-2.5Sn alloy using electric discharge machining process. Adv Mater Res 1137:39–51. https://doi.org/10.4028/WWW.SCIENTIFIC.NET/AMR.1137.39
35. Singh AK, Mahajan R, Tiwari A, Kumar D, Ghadai RK (2018) Effect of dielectric on electrical discharge machining: a review. IOP Conf Ser Mater Sci Eng 377. https://doi.org/10.1088/1757-899X/377/1/012184
36. Kumar R, Singh S, Bilga PS, Jatin, Singh J, Singh S, Scutaru ML, Pruncu CI (2021) Revealing the benefits of entropy weights method for multi-objective optimization in machining operations: a critical review. J Mater Res Technol 10:1471–1492. https://doi.org/10.1016/J.JMRT.2020.12.114
37. Philip JT, Kumar D, Mathew J, Kuriachen B (2020) Experimental investigations on the tribological performance of electric discharge alloyed Ti–6Al–4V at 200–600 °C. J Tribol 142. https://doi.org/10.1115/1.4046016/1072630
38. Chen YF, Lin YC (2009) Surface modifications of Al–Zn–Mg alloy using combined EDM with ultrasonic machining and addition of TiC particles into the dielectric. J Mater Process Technol 209:4343–4350. https://doi.org/10.1016/J.JMATPROTEC.2008.11.013

39. Yang TS, Huang MS, Wang MS, Lin MH, Tsai MY, Wang PYW (2013) Effect of electrical discharging on formation of nanoporous biocompatible layer on Ti–6Al–4V alloys. Implant Dent 22:374–379. https://doi.org/10.1097/ID.0B013E31829A170A
40. Lee WF, Yang TS, Wu YC, Peng PW (2013) Nanoporous biocompatible layer on Ti–6Al–4V alloys enhanced osteoblast-like cell response. J Exp Clin Med 5:92–96. https://doi.org/10.1016/J.JECM.2013.04.002
41. Murali M, Yeo SH (2004) Rapid biocompatible micro device fabrication by micro electro-discharge machining. Biomed Microdevices 6:41–45. https://doi.org/10.1023/B:BMMD.0000013364.71148.51
42. Mahmud N, Yahya A, Rafiq M, Samion S, Safura NL (2012) Electrical discharge machining pulse power generator to machine micropits of hip implant. In: 2012 international conference on biomedical engineering, ICoBE 2012, pp 493–497. https://doi.org/10.1109/ICOBE.2012.6179066
43. Klocke F, Schwade M, Klink A, Veselovac D, Kopp A (2013) Influence of electro discharge machining of biodegradable magnesium on the biocompatibility. Procedia CIRP 5:88–93. https://doi.org/10.1016/J.PROCIR.2013.01.018
44. Zinelis S, Al Jabbari YS, Thomas A, Silikas N, Eliades G (2013) Multitechnique characterization of CPTi surfaces after electro discharge machining (EDM). Clin Oral Investig 18(1):67–75. https://doi.org/10.1007/S00784-013-0962-Y
45. Bhui AS, Singh G, Sidhu SS, Bains PS (2018) Experimental investigation of optimal ED machining parameters for Ti–6Al–4V biomaterial. Facta Univ Ser Mech Eng 16:337–345. https://doi.org/10.22190/FUME180824033B
46. Shin KR, Kim YS, Jeong JH, Ko YG, Shin DH (2016) Pore size effect on cell response via plasma electrolytic oxidation. Surf Eng 32:418–422. https://doi.org/10.1179/1743294415Y.0000000026
47. Peng PW, Ou KL, Lin HC, Pan YN, Wang CH (2010) Effect of electrical-discharging on formation of nanoporous biocompatible layer on titanium. J Alloys Compd 492:625–630. https://doi.org/10.1016/J.JALLCOM.2009.11.197
48. Chang-Bin T, Dao-Xin L, Zhan W, Yang G (2011) Electro-spark alloying using graphite electrode on titanium alloy surface for biomedical applications. Appl Surf Sci 257:6364–6371. https://doi.org/10.1016/J.APSUSC.2011.01.120
49. Mahajan A, Devgan S, Sidhu SS (2021) Surface alteration of biomedical alloys by electrical discharge treatment for enhancing the electrochemical corrosion, tribological and biological performances. Surf Coat Technol 405:126583. https://doi.org/10.1016/J.SURFCOAT.2020.126583
50. Mahajan A, Sidhu SS, Devgan S (2020) Examination of hemocompatibility and corrosion resistance of electrical discharge-treated duplex stainless steel (DSS-2205) for biomedical applications. Appl Phys A 126(9):1–11. https://doi.org/10.1007/S00339-020-03940-5
51. Mahajan A, Singh G, Devgan S, Sidhu SS (2020) EDM performance characteristics and electrochemical corrosion analysis of Co–Cr alloy and duplex stainless steel: a comparative study. Proc Inst Mech Eng Part E J Process Mech Eng 235:812–823. https://doi.org/10.1177/0954408920976739
52. Ablyaz TR, Shlykov ES, Muratov KR, Mahajan A, Singh G, Devgan S, Sidhu SS (2020) Surface characterization and tribological performance analysis of electric discharge machined duplex stainless steel. Micromachines 11:926. https://doi.org/10.3390/MI11100926
53. Xu B, Lian MQ, Chen SG, Lei JG, Wu XY, Guo C, Peng TJ, Yang J, Luo F, Zhao H (2021) Combining PMEDM with the tool electrode sloshing to reduce recast layer of titanium alloy generated from EDM. Int J Adv Manuf Technol 117(5):1535–1545. https://doi.org/10.1007/S00170-021-07808-7
54. Elaiyarasan U, Satheeshkumar V, Senthilkumar C, Nandakumar C (2022) Mathematical and artificial neural network model in composite electrode assisted electrical discharge coating. Surf Topogr Metrol Prop 10:025004. https://doi.org/10.1088/2051-672X/AC63D7
55. Huang TS, Hsieh SF, Chen SL, Lin MH, Ou SF, Chang WT (2015) Surface modification of TiNi-based shape memory alloys by dry electrical discharge machining. J Mater Process Technol 221:279–284. https://doi.org/10.1016/J.JMATPROTEC.2015.02.025

56. Li L, Zhao L, Li ZY, Feng L, Bai X (2016) Surface characteristics of Ti–6Al–4V by SiC abrasive-mixed EDM with magnetic stirring. Mater Manuf Process 32:83–86. https://doi.org/10.1080/10426914.2016.1151043
57. Chen SL, Lin MH, Huang GX, Wang CC (2014) Research of the recast layer on implant surface modified by micro-current electrical discharge machining using deionized water mixed with titanium powder as dielectric solvent. Appl Surf Sci 311:47–53. https://doi.org/10.1016/J.APSUSC.2014.04.204
58. Bui VD, Mwangi JW, Schubert A (2019) Powder mixed electrical discharge machining for antibacterial coating on titanium implant surfaces. J Manuf Process 44:261–270. https://doi.org/10.1016/J.JMAPRO.2019.05.032
59. Sales WF, Oliveira ARF, Raslan AA (2016) Titanium perovskite ($CaTiO_3$) formation in Ti6Al4V alloy using the electrical discharge machining process for biomedical applications. Surf Coat Technol 307:1011–1015. https://doi.org/10.1016/J.SURFCOAT.2016.10.028
60. Prakash C, Singh S, Pruncu CI, Mishra V, Królczyk G, Pimenov DY, Pramanik A (2019) Surface modification of Ti–6Al–4V alloy by electrical discharge coating process using partially sintered Ti-Nb electrode. Materials 12:1006. https://doi.org/10.3390/MA12071006
61. Sharma G, Kumar K, Satsangi PS, Sharma N (2021) Surface modification of biodegradable Mg–4Zn alloy using PMEDM: an experimental investigation, optimization and corrosion analysis. IRBM. https://doi.org/10.1016/J.IRBM.2021.02.003
62. Razak MAHA, Abdul-Rani AM, Aliyu AAA (2019) Innovative surface engineering technique for surface modification of Mg alloy for orthopedic application. Biomanufacturing 225–240. https://doi.org/10.1007/978-3-030-13951-3_11/COVER/
63. Prakash C, Kansal HK, Pabla BS, Puri S (2017) On the influence of nanoporous layer fabricated by PMEDM on β-Ti implant: biological and computational evaluation of bone-implant interface. Mater Today Proc 4:2298–2307. https://doi.org/10.1016/J.MATPR.2017.02.078
64. Sadat-Shojai M, Khorasani MT, Dinpanah-Khoshdargi E, Jamshidi A (2013) Synthesis methods for nanosized hydroxyapatite with diverse structures. Acta Biomater 9:7591–7621. https://doi.org/10.1016/J.ACTBIO.2013.04.012
65. Öpöz TT, Yaşar H, Murphy MF, Ekmekci N, Ekmekci B (2019) Ti6Al4V surface modification by hydroxyapatite powder mixed electrical discharge machining for medical applications. Int J Adv Eng Pure Sci 31:1–10. https://doi.org/10.7240/JEPS.450383
66. Singh G, Sidhu SS, Bains PS, Singh M, Bhui AS (2020) On surface modification of Ti alloy by electro discharge coating using hydroxyapatite powder mixed dielectric with graphite tool. J Bio- Tribo-Corros 6(3):1–11. https://doi.org/10.1007/S40735-020-00389-0
67. Yaşar H, Ekmekci B (2021) The effect of micro and nano hydroxyapatite powder on biocompatibility and surface integrity of Ti6Al4V (ELI) in powder mixed electrical discharge machining. Surf Topogr Metrol Prop 9:015015. https://doi.org/10.1088/2051-672X/ABDDA2
68. Lamichhane Y, Singh G, Bhui AS, Mukhiya P, Kumar P, Thapa B (2019) Surface modification of 316L SS with HAp nano-particles using PMEDM for enhanced biocompatibility. Mater Today Proc 15:336–343. https://doi.org/10.1016/J.MATPR.2019.05.014
69. Arun Pillai KV, Hariharan P (2021) Experimental investigation on the recast layer and performance indicators during nano powder mixed μED milling of Ti–6Al–4V. Surf Topogr Metrol Prop 9:025041. https://doi.org/10.1088/2051-672X/AC0A39
70. Li X, Liu X, Huang J, Fan Y, Cui FZ (2011) Biomedical investigation of CNT based coatings. Surf Coat Technol 206:759–766. https://doi.org/10.1016/J.SURFCOAT.2011.02.063
71. Al-Amin M, Abdul-Rani AM, Rao TVVLN, Danish M, Rubaiee S, bin Mahfouz A, Parameswari RP, Wani MF (2022) Investigation of machining and modified surface features of 316L steel through novel hybrid of HA/CNT added-EDM process. Mater Chem Phys 276:125320. https://doi.org/10.1016/J.MATCHEMPHYS.2021.125320
72. Devgan S, Sidhu SS (2020) Potential of electrical discharge treatment incorporating MWCNTs to enhance the corrosion performance of the β-titanium alloy. Appl Phys A 126(3):1–16. https://doi.org/10.1007/S00339-020-3391-1
73. Devgan S, Mahajan A, Sidhu SS (2021) Multi-walled carbon nanotubes in powder mixed electrical discharge machining: an experimental study, state of the art and feasibility prospect. Appl Phys A 127(11):1–15. https://doi.org/10.1007/S00339-021-04934-7

Chapter 4
Electric Discharge Treatment of Co–Cr Alloy

This chapter provides an in-depth examination of the systematic experiments carried out on cobalt-chromium (Co–Cr) alloy substrates utilizing the electrical discharge coating (EDC) technique. The primary aim of this research is to analyze the impact of various electrical discharge machining (EDM) parameters on the surface properties, biocompatibility, and wear resistance of Co–Cr implants employed in biomedical applications. The specific alloy under investigation, ASTM F75, is widely recognized for its application in orthopedic and dental implants due to its excellent mechanical strength, durability, and inherent chemical inertness. These attributes make it suitable for long-term implantation in the human body. However, there remains a significant opportunity to enhance its surface characteristics, which in turn could optimize biological responses, including corrosion resistance, hemocompatibility, and cytocompatibility, factors that are critical in ensuring the longevity and effectiveness of implants. To achieve these goals, the research was structured around a comprehensive three-stage experimental approach. In the first stage, the baseline properties of the Co–Cr alloy were established, assessing parameters such as initial surface roughness and mechanical strength. The second stage involved the application of the EDC technique with varying EDM parameters, including discharge current, pulse duration, and electrode material, to modify the surface characteristics systematically. In the final stage, extensive evaluations of biocompatibility and wear behavior were conducted through a series of in-vitro and in-vivo tests, with the aim of determining how these modified surfaces interacted with biological tissues and fluids. This detailed exploration aims to contribute valuable insights into how optimizing the surface properties of Co–Cr alloys can lead to improved performance of biomedical implants, ultimately enhancing patient outcomes.

- **Stage I**: In this initial stage, there is an evaluation of the surface roughness and biological responses to different conditions by utilizing a full factorial design. This approach allows us to examine the effects of varying levels of current and pulse on-time simultaneously, providing a comprehensive understanding of how

© The Author(s), under exclusive license to Springer Nature Singapore Pte Ltd. 2026
A. Mahajan et al., *Surface Modification of Co–Cr Alloy for Orthopaedic Applications*, Biomedical Materials for Multi-functional Applications,
https://doi.org/10.1007/978-981-95-4029-7_4

these parameters influence the surface characteristics and biological compatibility of the materials being tested.

- **Stage II**: The second stage focuses on multi-parameter optimization. We employed a Taguchi L18 orthogonal array method, which enables us to efficiently assess a broad range of variables. This includes experimenting with multiple types of electrodes, various dielectric fluids, and different spark conditions. By carefully analyzing the interactions between these factors, we aim to identify the optimal combination that enhances performance while maintaining safety and efficacy.
- **Stage III**: In the final stage, we performed advanced biological and tribological testing. This will be conducted under the optimal electrical discharge machining (EDC) parameters identified in the earlier stages. The testing will focus on assessing the biological responses, such as cell viability and response, alongside tribological characteristics, including wear resistance and friction. This comprehensive analysis aims to ensure that the selected parameters not only improve the material properties but also meet the necessary biological standards for application.

4.1 Experimental Framework

A detailed experimental workflow was crafted (refer to Fig. 4.1) to thoroughly explore the influences of spark energy and the dielectric environment on both surface quality and biological responses. The study employed a die-sinking EDM, specifically the S645 CMAX model manufactured by OSCARMAX in Taiwan. This sophisticated machine operates based on the principle of spark erosion, which removes material from the workpiece through the precise application of high-frequency electrical discharges within a dielectric medium. To optimize the machining process, negative polarity was utilized, whereby the workpiece functioned as the cathode and the tool served as the anode. This arrangement is known to enhance material deposition and allows for controlled melting on the surface of the substrate, resulting in improved surface characteristics. In addition to the operational details, the experimental setup has been visually represented in Fig. 4.2, which illustrates the arrangement of equipment and the various components involved in the EDM process (see Table 4.1). This comprehensive approach not only aims to elucidate the relationship between spark energy and dielectric conditions but also seeks to provide insights into how these factors impact the biological responses of the treated materials.

4.2 Workpiece Material: ASTM F75 Co–Cr Alloy

The selected alloy adheres to ASTM F75 standards and is widely used in joint prostheses, particularly in the construction of hip and knee implants. This alloy was procured from DePuy Synthes, a reputable manufacturer known for its high-quality

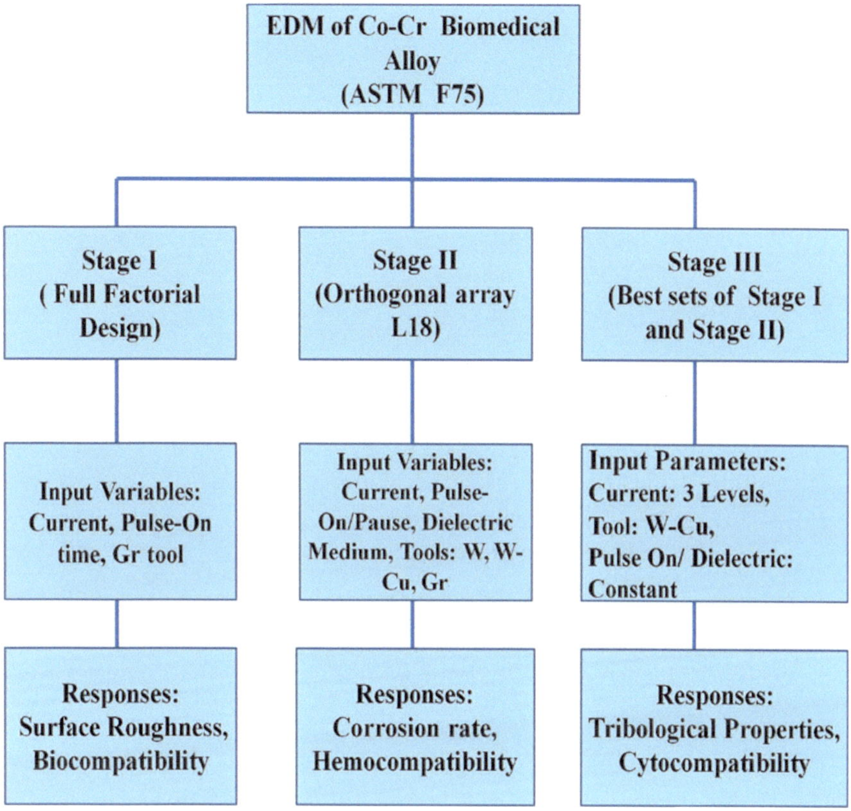

Fig. 4.1 Outline of the experimental approach

orthopedic materials in the USA. The primary component of the alloy is cobalt, which is strategically alloyed with chromium, molybdenum, and trace elements such as nickel, iron, and carbon (as detailed in Table 4.2). These elements work together to enhance the alloy's mechanical properties, offering exceptional tensile strength and durability, along with remarkable resistance to oxidative degradation. This combination not only ensures long-term performance in-vivo but also promotes compatibility with biological environments, reducing the risk of adverse reactions following implantation [1]. To better understand the microstructural characteristics of the femoral component, scanning electron microscopy (SEM) was employed, as illustrated in Fig. 4.3. The analysis revealed a fine-grain morphology and a detailed surface texture, both crucial for optimal integration with surrounding bone tissue. These microstructural features play a significant role in the alloy's overall performance in load-bearing applications. Furthermore, Table 4.3 presents comprehensive data on the alloy's mechanical properties, highlighting a tensile strength that exceeds 900 MPa and a Rockwell hardness of around 34 HRC. This level of hardness is particularly important for load-bearing implant applications, ensuring that the prosthesis

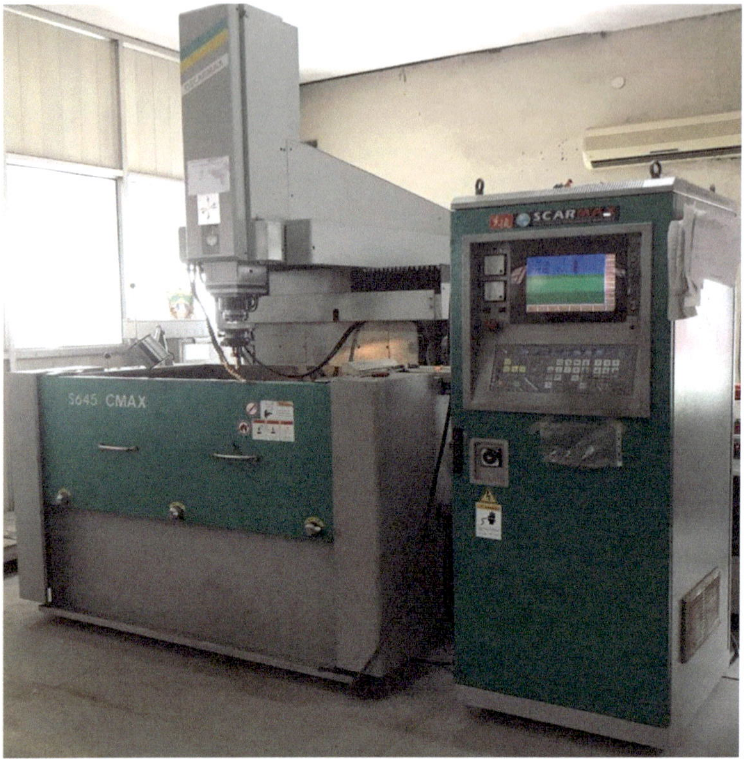

Fig. 4.2 Pictorial view of electrical discharge machining (model—S645 CMAX)

Table 4.1 Specification of EDM (model—S645 CMAX)

Parameters	Descriptions/value
Process mechanism	Spark erosion principle
Gap between spindle and worktable (mm)	355–755
Max weight of workpiece (kg)	3000
Max weight of electrode (kg)	250
Main table transverse (*X*, *Y*) (mm)	600, 450
Generator	EMS 5030
Interpolation	Linear and circular
Input power supply (kVA)	3 phase, AC 415 V, 50 Hz
Fluid tank capacity (L)	964
Tool materials	Copper, graphite, tungsten, brass, etc.
Dielectric fluid	EDM oil, kerosene oil, deionized water, etc.

can withstand the significant stresses experienced during normal activities without compromising its structural integrity [2].

Table 4.2 Chemical composition of cobalt-chromium (Co–Cr) alloy

	Cr	Mo	Si	Mn	Ni	C	Fe	Ti	P	Co
Base material	28.5%	6%	0.7%	0.5%	0.25%	0.22%	0.2%	0.01%	0.02%	Remainder

Reproduced with permission from Taylor & Francis [3]

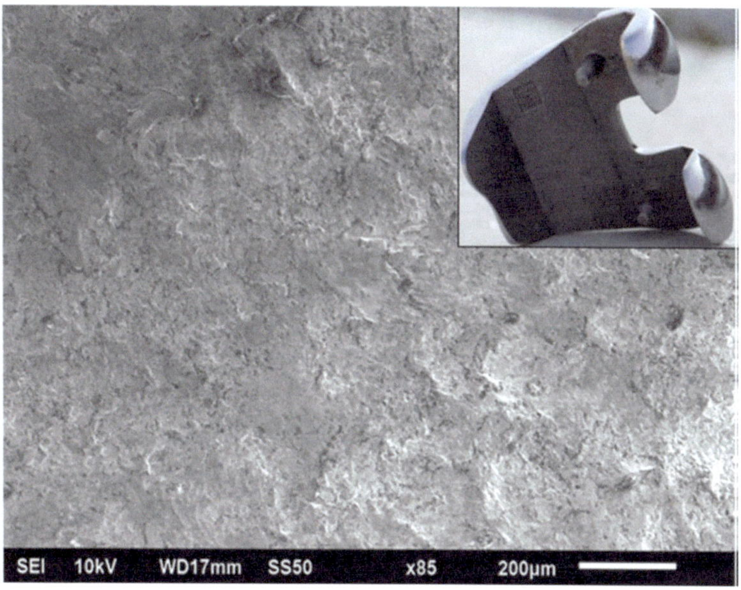

Fig. 4.3 SEM image and pictorial view (insert) of the femoral component of the knee joint. Reproduced with permission from Taylor & Francis [3]

Table 4.3 Mechanical properties of Co–Cr (ASTM F75) alloy

Properties	Values
Rockwell hardness (HRC)	34
Tensile strength (MPa)	920
Elongation (%)	16.5
Reduction of area (%)	20
Young's modulus (GPa)	216
Density (g/cm^3)	8.3

Reproduced with permission from Elsevier [2]

4.3 Variants Electrode Tool Employed for Experimental Work

Three types of electrodes were selected for their exceptional thermal, electrical, and biocompatibility characteristics, which make them suitable for a variety of applications:

- **Graphite**: Known for its outstanding machinability, graphite can be easily shaped and refined into precise electrode configurations. With a remarkably high melting point of about 3300 °C, it is highly resistant to thermal degradation. Additionally, graphite is chemically inert, meaning it does not react with other substances, which contributes to its stability and longevity in various environments. Its proven compatibility with biomedical surfaces makes it an ideal choice for applications in medical devices and implants [4–6].
- **Tungsten (W)**: Tungsten was selected for its exceptional hardness and impressive erosion resistance, properties that ensure durability and longevity in harsh operational conditions. This metal maintains dimensional stability under prolonged electrical discharges, which is crucial in applications that involve consistent electrical loads. Tungsten's high melting point further contributes to its suitability for high-temperature applications, making it a reliable choice in environments where other materials might degrade [7–9].
- **Tungsten-Copper (W–Cu, 75/25)**: This hybrid composite combines the advantageous properties of tungsten and copper, enhancing the performance of electrodes. Tungsten provides excellent heat resistance, allowing the electrode to withstand high temperatures without loss of integrity. In contrast, copper contributes superior electrical conductivity and low resistivity, which is vital for efficient electrical performance. The combination of these materials results in an electrode that performs well in both thermal and electrical applications, making it a versatile option for a range of advanced technological uses [10–12].

Figure 4.4 provides a detailed illustration of the physical design of electrodes, each measuring 10 mm in diameter. This specific size is crucial for optimizing performance in various EDM applications. In conjunction with this illustration, Table 4.4 presents a comprehensive summary of the thermal and electrical properties of these electrodes, including conductivity, thermal resistance, and melting points. These properties significantly influence two key aspects of EDM operations: the material removal rate, which determines the efficiency of the machining process, and the deposition characteristics, which affect the quality of the surfaces produced. Understanding the interplay between these factors is essential for selecting the appropriate electrode materials to achieve desired machining outcomes effectively.

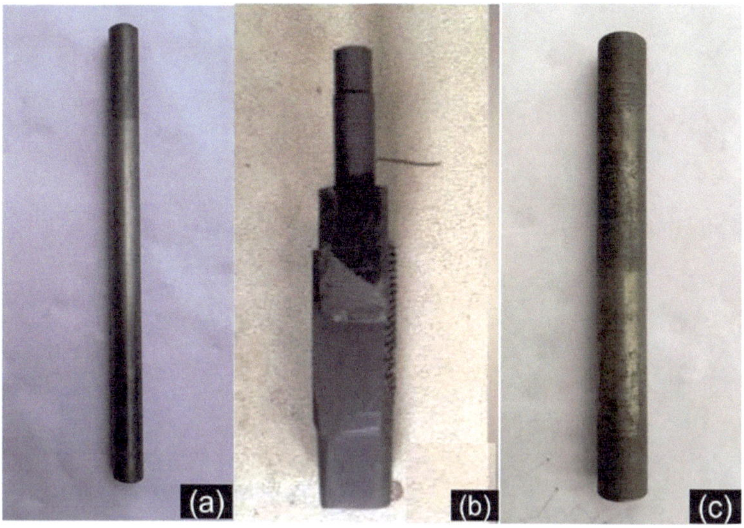

Fig. 4.4 Variants tool electrode employed for Stage II experimental work; **a** tungsten; **b** graphite; **c** tungsten-Cu (W/Cu-75/25) (diameter: 10 mm)

Table 4.4 Imperative properties of various electrodes

Electrodes	Essential properties			
	Melting range (°C)	Hardness (HB)	Density (g/cm^3)	Electrical resistivity (Ω cm)
Graphite	3300	10	1.77	1400
Tungsten	3400	2570	18.8	0.0001085
Tungsten–copper (W/Cu-75/25)	3410	195	14.5	4.5

Reproduced with permission from Elsevier [12]

4.4 Stage I: Full Factorial Design for Surface Roughness and Biocompatibility

The initial experiments were designed to thoroughly investigate the effects of two critical variables, current (I) and pulse on-time (P_{on}), on both surface quality and biological outcomes. By varying these parameters, we aimed to gain insights into how they influence the characteristics of the material's surface and the subsequent biological responses. The total spark energy imparted during these processes is calculated using Eq. 4.1, which serves as a key determinant in understanding the overall effectiveness of the treatment. This equation not only reflects the energy dynamics involved but also allows us to correlate the changes in surface quality with measurable biological responses, thereby enhancing our understanding of the relationship

Table 4.5 Parameter descriptions and values for Stage I

Parameter, units	Values
Current (I), A	1, 5, 10, 16
On-time (P_{on}), μs	20, 60, 150, 200

Reproduced with permission from Taylor & Francis [3]

between these factors.

$$E = V \times I \times P_{\text{on}} \tag{4.1}$$

where E is energy in joules (J); V is voltage (140 V constant); I is current (1–16 A); P_{on} is pulse on-time (20–200 μs).

Table 4.5 provides a comprehensive overview of the process parameters and their corresponding levels employed during the experimental stage of the study. In this phase, a full factorial design was carried out, resulting in 16 distinct combinations of variables, which are detailed in Table 4.6. To assess the quality of the machining process, surface roughness was meticulously measured using profilometry, a precise method that evaluates the texture of the machined surfaces. Following this, biological responses were evaluated through standard biomedical assays, focusing on key metrics such as the percentage of hemolysis and cell viability. These assays are critical for understanding the biocompatibility of the materials involved, ensuring they are suitable for potential medical applications.

Table 4.6 Full factorial experimental array of Stage I

Trial No.	I (A)	P_{on} (μs)	Responses
1	1	20	Surface roughness (μm), % hemolysis and % cell viability
2	1	60	
3	1	150	
4	1	200	
5	5	20	
6	5	60	
7	5	150	
8	5	200	
9	10	20	
10	10	60	
11	10	150	
12	10	200	
13	16	20	
14	16	60	
15	16	150	
16	16	200	

4.5 Stage II: Multi-parameter Optimization Using Taguchi Design

To effectively account for the numerous variables that can influence EDC outcomes, the research methodology employed a Taguchi L18 orthogonal array during the second stage of experimentation. This sophisticated statistical approach is designed to facilitate the efficient testing of five different factors while minimizing the number of experimental runs required. By systematically varying these factors, we can better understand their individual and collective effects on EDC outcomes. For further clarity, Table 4.7 details the specific process parameters and their corresponding levels utilized throughout the experiments, providing a comprehensive overview of the experimental setup.

The selection of dielectric fluid played a critical role in the machining process. In this context, EDM oil is known for its excellent insulation properties and low viscosity, which help to ensure consistent electrical contact and precision during machining. Conversely, deionized water is favored for its superior cooling capabilities, which can lead to more effective temperature management during operations and subsequently contribute to reduced tool wear and increased tool longevity. In Table 4.8, we present the experimental design, specifically the L18 layout, along with the various test conditions applied throughout the study. Following the machining process, each sample was sectioned to precise dimensions of 10 mm in diameter and 3 mm in thickness using wire-EDM techniques. This careful preparation was essential for ensuring accurate results in subsequent testing. To evaluate the corrosion resistance of the materials, we conducted potentiodynamic polarization testing, a technique that allows us to establish the electrochemical behavior of the samples in a controlled environment. Additionally, we assessed hemocompatibility by performing human red blood cell (RBC) lysis assays, which determines how the materials interact with human blood components, a crucial factor in applications involving medical devices or implants. This comprehensive approach ensures that we obtain a thorough understanding of both the physical and biological properties of the samples.

Table 4.7 Parameter descriptions and values for Stage II

Parameter, units	Values
Current (I), A	5, 10, 16
On-time (P_{on}), μs Pause time (P_{off}), μs	60, 150, 200 60, 150, 200
Electrode	Gr, W, W–Cu
Dielectric medium	EDM oil, deionized water

Reproduced with permission from Springer Nature [13]

Table 4.8 L18 experimental design layout and levels of Stage II

Trial No.	I (A)	P_{on} (μs)	P_{off} (μs)	Electrode	Dielectric medium	Responses
1	5	60	60	Gr	EDM oil	Corrosion rate (mm/year)
2	5	150	150	W	EDM oil	
3	5	200	200	W–Cu	EDM oil	
4	10	60	60	W	EDM oil	
5	10	150	150	W–Cu	EDM oil	
6	10	200	200	Gr	EDM oil	
7	16	60	150	Gr	EDM oil	
8	16	150	200	W	EDM oil	
9	16	200	60	W–Cu	EDM oil	
10	5	60	200	W–Cu	Deionized water	
11	5	150	60	Gr	Deionized water	
12	5	200	150	W	Deionized water	
13	10	60	150	W–Cu	Deionized water	
14	10	150	200	Gr	Deionized water	
15	10	200	60	W	Deionized water	
16	16	60	200	W	Deionized water	
17	16	150	60	W–Cu	Deionized water	
18	16	200	150	Gr	Deionized water	

Reproduced with permission from Springer Nature [13]

4.6 Stage III: Validation of Optimized Conditions

In Stage III of our experimentation, we aimed to investigate the application and effectiveness of EDM treatment on the substrate in order to enhance both the cytocompatibility and tribological properties of medical-grade cobalt-chromium (Co–Cr) alloy. This stage involved selecting the most promising EDM process outcomes from the earlier stages (Stages I and II), which provided critical insights essential for the development of metallic implants used in medical applications. For our experiments, the Co–Cr specimens were subjected to treatment using a tungsten-copper (W–Cu) electrode in a deionized water tank, which served as the dielectric medium. We conducted the treatment at various spark energy levels to assess how these different energy inputs would affect the material's properties. To evaluate the cytocompatibility of the treated substrates, we performed an MTT assay, a well-established method for measuring cell viability. This assay helps us determine how well cells can survive and proliferate on the treated surfaces, providing crucial information about the biological compatibility of the material for potential use in implants. Additionally, we evaluated the wear rate and coefficient of friction of the substrates using a pin-on-disk tribometer. This method allows us to simulate the conditions that the material would encounter in actual use, providing valuable data on its durability and performance under mechanical stress. By combining these analyses, we aimed to gain a comprehensive understanding of how electric discharge treatment can improve the properties of Co–Cr alloys for medical applications.

In this study, the previous stages (I and II) were utilized as critical resources for selecting appropriate machining parameters in Stage III, as depicted in Fig. 4.5. Specifically, we identified and selected EDM parameters from Stage II that exhibited remarkable corrosion resistance and hemocompatibility, essential qualities for the intended applications of the materials. The second sample was derived from the L18 experimental design established in Stage II, where we specifically focused on achieving spark energy that aligned with the bio-favorable range previously identified in Stage I. This careful selection ensures that the machining process supports optimal material performance in biological environments. For the third set of parameters, we opted for the lowest current while keeping the pulse on-time consistent with those used in the first and second samples. The use of deionized water as the dielectric medium further enhances the precision and effectiveness of the machining process. This selection of parameters is grounded in the findings from Stage II, guaranteeing that the final outcomes will meet stringent performance criteria.

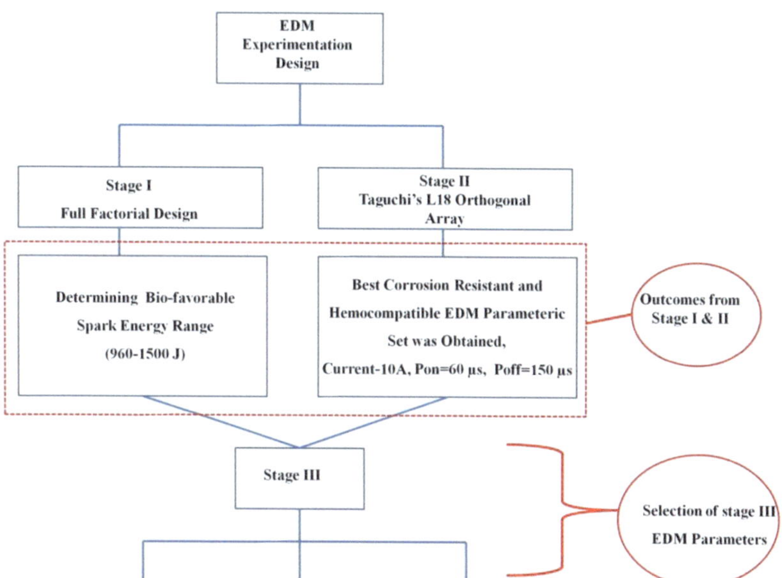

Input Factors	Trial 1	Trial 2	Trial 3
Current (A)	5	10	16
Pulse on Time (µs)	60	60	60
Pulse off Time(µs)	200	150	200
Voltage(V)	140		
Electrode	Tungsten Copper (W-Cu)		
Dielectric Medium	Deionized Water		

Fig. 4.5 Selection of Stage III EDM process parameters

4.7 Statistical Analysis

To evaluate the significance of various parameters in the study, a range of statistical tools was utilized. Specifically, Analysis of Variance (ANOVA) was implemented during both Stage I and Stage II to determine the primary factors affecting surface roughness and corrosion rate of the materials under investigation. The analysis was conducted at a rigorous 95% confidence level, where a p-value less than 0.05 was considered statistically significant. In this context, factors that exhibited higher F-values were identified as having a stronger influence on the measured outcomes, indicating their critical role in the performance of the materials. Conversely, factors associated with lower p-values were deemed statistically reliable, reaffirming their importance in the overall analysis. This comprehensive approach ensured a robust evaluation of the data, allowing for a clearer understanding of the relationships between the variables studied.

4.8 Advanced Characterization Techniques

To gain a comprehensive understanding of the physical and chemical transformations that occur after the electrical discharge coated surface, several advanced characterization tools were employed, each serving a specific purpose:

- **X-Ray Diffraction (XRD)**: This technique was instrumental in identifying the formation of new crystalline phases within the coated materials [14]. By analyzing the diffraction patterns, we could determine the surface crystallinity, which provides insights into the structural integrity and potential mechanical properties of the coated surface [15, 16].
- **Scanning Electron Microscopy (SEM)**: SEM allowed for an in-depth morphological analysis of the coated surfaces. This method revealed critical details regarding deposition quality, including uniformity and coverage, as well as the porosity of the coatings, which can affect their performance and durability. Furthermore, SEM was utilized to examine the wear characteristics of the materials, revealing how the coatings performed under simulated operational conditions. In addition, the technique was used to assess the hemocompatibility of the coatings through the analysis of red blood cell (RBC) interactions, which is crucial for applications in biomedical devices. The corrosion behavior of both the EDM-treated and untreated samples was also evaluated using SEM, facilitating comparisons between the two [17, 18].
- **Energy Dispersive X-Ray Spectroscopy (EDX)**: This analytical method complemented the SEM analysis by confirming the elemental composition of the coatings. EDX provided valuable data regarding the deposition of specific elements, particularly tungsten and copper, derived from the tool electrodes. This information is essential for understanding the mechanisms behind coating adhesion and overall material performance. Together, these advanced characterization techniques offer

a thorough examination of the coatings, revealing their structural, morphological, and compositional properties, which are critical for optimizing their performance in various applications [19, 20].

4.9 Conclusions

This chapter provides an in-depth exploration of experimental work conducted on cobalt-chromium (Co–Cr) alloy using the electrical discharge coating process, aimed at improving the surface properties of the alloy for medical implant applications. The significance of this study lies in its ability to enhance the biocompatibility and wear resistance of Co–Cr alloys, which are commonly used in orthopedic and dental implants. The study begins by identifying critical process parameters that influence the EDC process, such as discharge current, pulse duration, and the composition of the dielectric fluid. An experimental matrix is then designed to systematically assess the effects of these parameters on the quality and performance of the coated surfaces. The experimentation is structured into three distinct stages: (i) The first stage involves performing EDM treatment using a full factorial design, which allows for a comprehensive analysis of all possible combinations of the identified process parameters. This approach ensures that the interactions between different variables are thoroughly examined. (ii) The second stage focuses on optimizing the process parameters through the application of an L18 orthogonal array. This technique simplifies the optimization process by reducing the number of experiments needed while still providing valuable insights into the most effective parameter combinations. (iii) In the final stage, the best-performing EDM-treated specimens are subjected to rigorous evaluations to measure their tribological (friction and wear) and biological (cell compatibility and interaction) performance, ensuring their suitability for use in medical applications.

The chapter further elaborates on the experimental setup, detailing the specific materials used, including the substrates and electrode types, as well as the machining conditions applied during the process. It also highlights the methods for response evaluations, ensuring a comprehensive understanding of data collection. To provide a robust analysis, the chapter incorporates statistical methods alongside characterization techniques such as scanning electron microscopy (SEM) for assessing surface morphology, X-ray diffraction (XRD) for determining phase composition, and energy dispersive X-ray spectroscopy (EDX) for chemical analysis. Together, these techniques offer valuable insights into how the EDM process affects the microstructural and chemical properties of the Co–Cr alloy, ultimately supporting its application in both orthopedic and dental fields. This detailed examination aims to lay the groundwork for future advancements in the development of high-performance medical implants.

References

1. Hyslop DJS, Abdelkader AM, Cox A, Fray DJ (2010) Electrochemical synthesis of a biomedically important Co–Cr alloy. Acta Mater 58(8):3124–3130
2. Baron S, Ahearne E (2018) Fundamental mechanisms of chip formation in orthogonal cutting of medical grade cobalt chromium alloy (ASTM F75). CIRP J Manuf Sci Technol 23:54–63
3. Mahajan A, Sidhu SS (2018) Enhancing biocompatibility of Co–Cr alloy implants via electrical discharge process. Mater Technol 33(8):524–531
4. Beri N, Maheshwari S, Sharma C, Kumar A (2010) Technological advancement in electrical discharge machining with powder metallurgy processed electrodes: a review. Mater Manuf Process 25(10):1186–1197
5. Mahajan A, Sidhu SS, Ablyaz T (2019) EDM surface treatment: an enhanced biocompatible interface. In: Biomaterials in orthopaedics and bone regeneration: design and synthesis. Springer Singapore, Singapore, pp 33–40
6. Yadav R, Sharma AK, Sharma S (2025) Advance development in natural graphite material and its applications: a review. Min Metall Explor 42(1):361–385
7. Bhaumik M, Maity K (2019) Effect of electrode materials on different EDM aspects of titanium alloy. Silicon 11(1):187–196
8. Hossain A, Manu R, Shibli SMA (2023) Chemically modified carbon nanotubes for tribology applications. In: Chemically modified carbon nanotubes for commercial applications, pp 441–461
9. Barua A, Pradhan S, Priyadarshini M, Patra A, Kumari K (2024) Recent advancement in tungsten heavy alloy processing for different industrial applications. J Mater Eng Perform 1–21
10. Zhang B, Yang K, Huang Z, Wang J (2024) Recent advances in W–Cu composites: a review on the fabrication, application, property, densification, and strengthening mechanism. Adv Eng Mater 26(1):2301204
11. Omole S, Lunt A, Kirk S, Shokrani A (2022) Advanced processing and machining of tungsten and its alloys. J Manuf Mater Process 6(1):15
12. Jahan MP, Wong YS, Rahman M (2009) A study on the fine-finish die-sinking micro-EDM of tungsten carbide using different electrode materials. J Mater Process Technol 209(8):3956–3967
13. Mahajan A, Sidhu SS (2019) In vitro corrosion and hemocompatibility evaluation of electrical discharge treated cobalt–chromium implant. J Mater Res 34(8):1363–1370
14. Khan H, Yerramilli AS, D'Oliveira A, Alford TL, Boffito DC, Patience GS (2020) Experimental methods in chemical engineering: X-ray diffraction spectroscopy—XRD. Can J Chem Eng 98(6):1255–1266
15. Thakur A, Kumar A, Kaya S, Marzouki R, Zhang F, Guo L (2022) Recent advancements in surface modification, characterization and functionalization for enhancing the biocompatibility and corrosion resistance of biomedical implants. Coatings 12(10):1459
16. Gong F, Zhang J, Ding L, Yang Z, Liu X (2017) Mussel-inspired coating of energetic crystals: a compact core–shell structure with highly enhanced thermal stability. Chem Eng J 309:140–150
17. Giurlani W, Berretti E, Innocenti M, Lavacchi A (2020) Measuring the thickness of metal coatings: a review of the methods. Coatings 10(12):1211
18. Gautam K, Gogoi D, Kongnyui TD, Devi S, Kumar C, Kumar M (2024) A comprehensive review on surface modifications of polymer-based 3D-printed structures: metal coating prospects and challenges. Polym Adv Technol 35(4):e6369
19. Moridi A, Hassani-Gangaraj SM, Guagliano M, Dao M (2014) Cold spray coating: review of material systems and future perspectives. Surf Eng 30(6):369–395
20. Rezic I, Mestrovic E (2023) Characterization of nanoparticles in antimicrobial coatings for medical applications—a review. Coatings 13(11):1830

Chapter 5
In-Vitro Biocompatibility Analysis of EDMed Co–Cr Alloy (Stage I)

This chapter provides an in-depth analysis of the experimental investigations conducted on the machining of cobalt-chromium (Co–Cr) samples. The study explores the impact of various process control parameters, detailing how these can influence the outcomes of machining operations. The experimental responses were precisely recorded according to the designed experimental framework outlined in Chap. 4. Each phase of the research was examined in detail to ensure comprehensive coverage of the results. Key findings related to in-vitro biocompatibility are also methodically analyzed and discussed in this section. This includes an evaluation of how machining variables can affect the biological response of the Co–Cr samples, contributing valuable insights into their suitability for biomedical applications. The analysis not only highlights the significance of the machining parameters but also emphasizes the relationship between these parameters and the overall performance of Co–Cr materials in clinical settings.

5.1 Description of Stage I Experimentation

This phase of the study is dedicated to a comprehensive evaluation of the effects of EDM on the surface characteristics of medical-grade cobalt-chromium (Co–Cr) implants, which are widely used in orthopedic and dental applications due to their excellent biocompatibility and mechanical properties. To further explore the implications of these surface modifications, in-vitro tests were carried out to assess both cytocompatibility, how well cells interact with the material surfaces, and hemocompatibility, the interaction of the surfaces with blood components, aiming to provide insights into their biological interactions in a clinical setting. Initially, the Co–Cr implant material was sectioned into rectangular specimens to create uniform test samples. These specimens underwent a mechanical polishing process using silicon carbide emery paper of specified grade P1000. This step was crucial for achieving a

© The Author(s), under exclusive license to Springer Nature Singapore Pte Ltd. 2026

A. Mahajan et al., *Surface Modification of Co–Cr Alloy for Orthopaedic Applications*, Biomedical Materials for Multi-functional Applications,
https://doi.org/10.1007/978-981-95-4029-7_5

smooth surface finish, which is essential for accurate assessment of the EDM results. After polishing, the samples were thoroughly cleaned with ethanol to eliminate any contaminants that could affect the subsequent machining process and the integrity of the surface being analyzed. The EDM machining process was conducted using a die-sinking EDM setup, specifically designed for precision applications. This setup featured a fine graphite electrode with a particle size of approximately 5 μm, allowing for detailed and controlled machining of the implant surfaces. The EDM process was configured with negative polarity, meaning that the workpiece acted as the cathode (−) while the electrode functioned as the anode (+). This configuration plays a vital role in machining efficiency and the quality of the surface finish, ultimately affecting the material's performance in biological environments. By combining detailed manufacturing techniques with rigorous testing protocols, this study aims to provide a deeper understanding of how EDM influences the properties of Co–Cr implants, which could lead to improved outcomes in surgical applications.

5.1.1 Surface Roughness Evaluation

The surface roughness of the machined cobalt-chromium (Co–Cr) specimens was quantified at three distinct positions to ensure a comprehensive assessment, utilizing a surface profilometer (Model: Mitutoyo SJ-400) for accurate measurements. The primary metric employed in this analysis was the arithmetic mean roughness (Ra, in micrometers), which serves as an important indicator of the average deviation of the surface profile from the mean line. By focusing on Ra, we were able to effectively evaluate the degree of material erosion or deposition that occurred as a result of the electrical discharge machining process. To facilitate this measurement, the surface profilometer was meticulously set up in a controlled environment. Figure 5.1 illustrates the configuration of the surface profilometer, highlighting its key components and operational setup. This setup was essential for obtaining precise and reliable data. Additionally, the technical specifications of the surface roughness tester, which detail its capabilities and accuracy, are summarized in Table 5.1. This thorough investigation into surface roughness is crucial for understanding the material's performance characteristics and its suitability for various applications in engineering and biomedical fields.

5.1.2 Evaluation of Biological Response of EDMed Surface

To thoroughly evaluate the biological response of surfaces modified through EDM, we conducted a series of in-vitro tests, specifically focusing on hemolysis and cytocompatibility. Hemolysis tests help determine the potential of materials to cause the rupture of red blood cells, which is an important factor in assessing biocompatibility, while cytocompatibility tests measure how materials interact with living cells. Prior

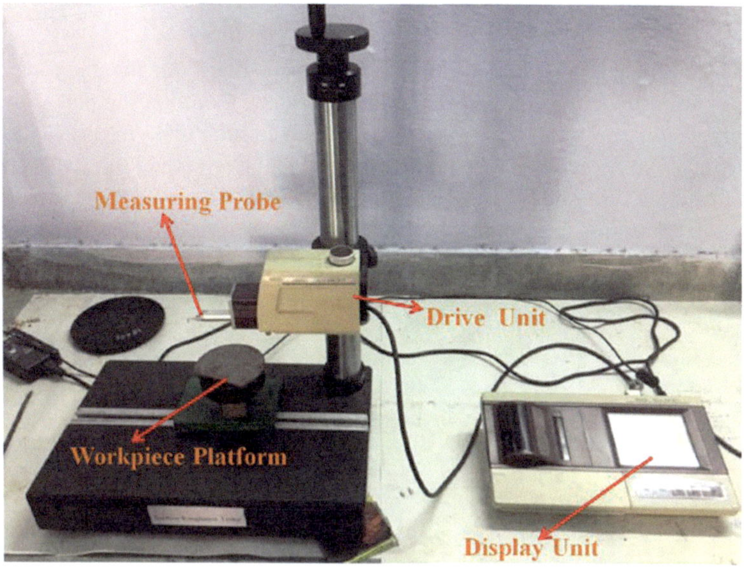

Fig. 5.1 Surface roughness tester (Mitutoyo SJ-400)

Table 5.1 Specification of surface roughness tester (SJ-400)

Parameters		Specification
Drive unit	Measuring range	25–50 mm
	Measuring speed	0.05, 0.1, 0.5, 1.0 mm/s
	Return speed	0.5, 1.0, 2.0 mm/s
Detector unit	Measurement method	Skidless/skidded
	Measuring force	4 mN or 0.75 mN
	Stylus tip	Diamond, 90°/5 μm R
	Measuring range/resolution	800 μm/0.000125 μm (at 8 μm range)
Data output		RS-232C interface/SPC output

to these tests, all samples underwent a rigorous sterilization procedure to ensure the removal of any contaminants and microorganisms that could interfere with the results. This was achieved using a moist heat sterilization method, specifically autoclaving, where the samples were subjected to a temperature of 121 °C for a duration of 20 min. This process was carried out using an autoclave unit (Narang Scientific Works, New Delhi, India). To ensure the accuracy and reliability of the findings, each test was replicated three times, allowing us to confirm consistency across the results and draw meaningful conclusions regarding the biological safety and compatibility of the EDMed-modified surfaces. This approach improves the potential applications of these surfaces in biomedical fields.

Hemocompatibility Test

After successfully completing the EDM process in line with the selected design matrix, an in-vitro hemolysis test was conducted on the modified samples to evaluate their hemocompatibility. The samples were cut into circular disks measuring 8 mm in diameter and 3 mm in thickness, enabling direct contact with red blood cells (RBCs). This contact was essential for assessing the potential for RBC lysis, which is a critical factor in determining the biocompatibility of the materials. For the hemocompatibility assessment, healthy human blood was obtained and collected in heparinized microcentrifuge tubes to prevent coagulation. The samples were centrifuged at a speed of 2500 rpm for 5 min at a temperature of 4 °C. This process effectively separated the RBCs from the other components present in the blood. Following centrifugation, the supernatant, which contained plasma and the buffy coat rich in leukocytes, was carefully removed. The RBC pellet underwent three washes with isotonic phosphate-buffered saline (PBS) at a pH of 7.4 to eliminate any remaining plasma proteins and contaminants. This washing step was crucial to ensure that the suspension used in the experiment consisted solely of isolated RBCs. Subsequently, a 1% RBC suspension was prepared from the washed pellet, which was then utilized in the study. This suspension allowed for accurate evaluation of the hemolytic potential of the modified samples, providing insight into their interactions with red blood cells and overall hemocompatibility. The schematic representation of the hemocompatibility test procedure is shown in Fig. 5.2.

The experimental samples were systematically arranged in 12-well plates, ensuring their modified (treated) surfaces were directly in contact with red blood cells (RBCs). Each well was filled with 1 ml of a 1% stock RBC suspension, providing a controlled environment for the hemolytic assessment. For the experimental setup, Triton from plate number 1 was utilized as the positive control; this agent is well-documented for inducing complete hemolysis (100%) of RBCs through membrane disruption. In contrast, isotonic PBS at pH 7.4 was employed as the negative control due to its known minimal hemolytic activity, allowing for effective comparison. The plates were incubated at a controlled temperature of 37 °C for one hour, providing optimal conditions for potential hemolysis to occur. Following the incubation period, the RBC suspensions in contact with the samples were carefully transferred into microcentrifuge tubes to avoid disturbing the samples. The centrifugation was conducted at 2500 rpm for 5 min at 4 °C to effectively separate the RBCs from the supernatant, allowing for the clear collection of the released hemoglobin. After centrifugation, the supernatant was carefully collected, and its absorbance was measured at 540 nm using a spectrophotometer. This wavelength is specific for detecting hemoglobin, enabling precise quantification of hemolysis [2]. The percentage of hemolysis was calculated using a standard formula (Eq. 5.1), which facilitated a detailed analysis of the hemolytic potential of the experimental samples compared to the established controls. This comprehensive approach allows for a clearer understanding of the interactions between the modified surfaces and the RBCs.

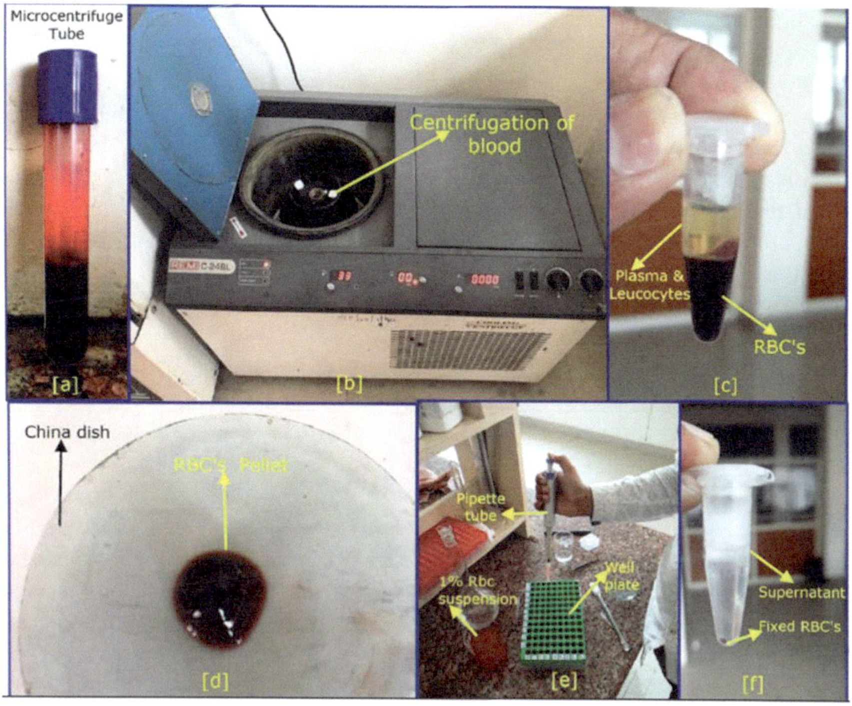

Fig. 5.2 **a** Blood accumulation in heparinized microcentrifuge tubes; **b** centrifugation of blood at 2500 rpm, 4 °C for 5 min; **c** separation of RBC's from plasma and leucocytes; **d** pellet of RBC's in China dish after washing with PBS; **e** preparation of 1% RBC suspension (mixture of RBC and PBS) and squeeze this suspension on Co–Cr samples with pipette tube in well plate; **f** final RBC pellet and supernatant obtained after incubation (37 °C, 1 h) as well as centrifugation (2500 rpm, 4 °C, 5 min). From the supernatant, the absorbance was computed, and to visualize RBC morphology under a microscope, the pellet was spread on a glass slide, and a coverslip was placed on it. Reproduced with permission from Springer Nature [1]

$$\%\,\text{hemolysis} = \frac{\text{ABs}}{\text{ABp}} * 100 \tag{5.1}$$

where ABs is the absorbance of testing samples, and ABp is the absorbance of the positive control.

Following a one-hour incubation period, the resulting pellet of RBCs was carefully re-suspended. To fix the cells, the suspension was treated with 0.5% glutaraldehyde in PBS at 4 °C for 1.5 h. This process ensures that the cellular structure is preserved for subsequent analysis. To eliminate any excess free glutaraldehyde that might interfere with the imaging process, the sample underwent centrifugation at 2000 rpm for 10 min, also at 4 °C. After centrifugation, the pellet was rinsed three times with distilled water to ensure thorough removal of the fixative, thus preparing the cells for accurate observation. The final RBC suspension was then prepared for SEM analysis. The analysis was conducted using an S-3400 microscope manufactured by

Hitachi Ltd. in Japan, operated at an acceleration voltage of 10 kV, which allows for high-resolution imaging of the cell surfaces. For the SEM imaging, samples were carefully mounted on carbon adhesive tape to secure them in place. To enhance the conductivity of the samples and improve image quality, they were sputter-coated with a gold–palladium alloy using the E-1010 coater from Hitachi Ltd. This coating not only enhances the electron emission during imaging but also prevents charging effects that can obscure details. Observations were made at various magnifications to capture a comprehensive view of RBC morphology, as detailed in the referenced literature [3].

Cytocompatibility Test

The cytocompatibility of the test samples was thoroughly evaluated using the MTT assay, which stands for 3-(4,5-dimethylthiazol-2-yl)-2,5-diphenyltetrazolium bromide (chemical formula: $C_{18}H_{16}BrN_5S$). This assay was conducted with two specific cell lines: MCF-7, which is a well-established human breast adenocarcinoma cell line, and HeLa, a widely used cervical cancer cell line. The testing was performed based on established protocols to ensure reliability and reproducibility. Camptothecin (CPT), at a concentration of 25 μM and sourced from Sigma located in Pune, India, was utilized as the positive control in the experiment. Its cytotoxic properties are well-documented in the literature, making it an appropriate comparison for measuring the effectiveness of the test samples. Conversely, Dulbecco's Modified Eagle Medium (DMEM) was employed as the negative control due to its proven capability to sustain 100% cell viability under standard laboratory conditions. The cells were cultured in DMEM, which was supplemented with 10% fetal bovine serum (FBS), essential for providing growth factors and nutrients, as well as 4500 mg/L of glucose to support cellular metabolism. Additionally, L-glutamine, sodium bicarbonate, and sodium pyruvate, all sourced from PAA Laboratories GmbH in Austria, were included in the medium to promote optimal cell growth and viability. Cultures were maintained in a controlled environment at 37 °C with 5% CO_2 for a period of 24 h. The use of a CO_2 incubator (Model HF100 from Heal Force, Shanghai, China) ensured stable conditions for cellular respiration and growth. This approach allows for an accurate assessment of the test sample cytocompatibility in comparison to both positive and negative controls.

Following the incubation period, cells were carefully seeded into 24-well plates (Thomas Scientific, Swedesboro, New Jersey, USA) at a specific density of 50,000 cells per well. Each well was equipped with a metal disk sample, precisely designed with a diameter of 8 mm and a thickness of 3 mm to ensure uniform exposure. After an exposure time of 48 h, the metal disks were systematically removed from each well. To assess cell viability, MTT solution was introduced at a concentration of 0.5 mg/ml (final concentration; Himedia, Mumbai, India). The plates were incubated for an additional 3 h, allowing viable cells to metabolize the MTT and reduce it to insoluble formazan crystals, which produced a distinct purple coloration. The formation of formazan is directly related to cell viability, and thus, its extent was measured and compared to standard positive and negative controls to validate the results. Once the incubation period was complete, the MTT solution was carefully aspirated to avoid disturbing the cells, and 1000 μl of dimethyl sulfoxide (DMSO) was added to each well. This step was crucial as DMSO served to dissolve the formazan crystals, facilitating accurate measurement. The absorbance of the resulting solution was measured at a wavelength of 570 nm using a spectrophotometer, providing quantitative data on cell viability. To ensure the reliability of the results, all experiments were conducted in triplicate [4]. The percentage of cell viability was then calculated using the established formula (Eq. 5.2), allowing for a comprehensive analysis of the effects of the metal disks on cellular health.

$$\%\,\text{Cell Viability} = \frac{\text{ABs}}{\text{ABc}} * 100 \tag{5.2}$$

where ABs is the absorbance of the testing samples, and ABc is the absorbance of the control.

5.2 Results and Discussion

The experimental findings demonstrate that the Co–Cr alloy, specifically the ASTM F75 grade, presents significant potential for application in the fabrication of orthopedic implants when processed using EDM. This advanced machining technique not only efficiently removes material but also enables concurrent surface modification, resulting in enhanced dimensional accuracy and improved clinical functionality. In this study, the Co–Cr biomedical alloy was machined with a fine-grained graphite electrode, which had a diameter of 10 mm. The machining process was conducted in the presence of a dielectric fluid, with options including either mineral oil or a specialized EDM fluid. The selection of these fluids is crucial, as they play a vital role in dielectric properties and effective flushing of debris during the machining process. To assess the influence of key machining parameters on the output characteristics of the machined surfaces, various variables were systematically varied. These included peak current and pulse-on duration, which are critical factors that can significantly affect the thermal and electrical dynamics during EDM. The study aimed to evaluate their impact particularly on two crucial aspects: surface roughness, which affects the biocompatibility and osseointegration of implants, and bioactivity, which determines the interaction between the implant surface and biological tissues. Through this comprehensive investigation, the research seeks to provide valuable insights into optimizing EDM parameters for enhancing the performance and longevity of orthopedic implants made from Co–Cr alloys.

5.2.1 Surface Roughness

The surface treatment process was executed in accordance with a pre-defined experimental matrix, as detailed in Table 5.2. This study focused on analyzing the surface texture resulting from the intricate phenomena of crater formation and the subsequent redeposition of material during the EDM process. To obtain reliable measurements, surface texture was quantified at five distinct locations on each sample, ensuring a comprehensive assessment. The average roughness values from these locations are summarized in the final column of Table 5.2. A detailed analysis of the surface roughness data collected from various trials revealed that the peak current plays a crucial role in influencing the machining outcomes. This relationship was statistically validated through an ANOVA test, which yielded a p-value of less than 0.05, indicating strong significance in the findings. Figure 5.3 provides a visual representation of how surface roughness varies in response to different EDM parameters, allowing for a clearer understanding of the relationships involved. Throughout the experiments, a finely finished surface exhibiting an average roughness (Ra) of 0.42 μm was successfully achieved when operating under a current of 10 A and a pulse-on time of 60 μs. This specific combination of parameters led to enhanced surface smoothness, which is often desirable in precision machining applications. Conversely, the roughest surface recorded during the trials had an Ra of 2.47 μm, occurring at a higher current of 16 A combined with a pulse-on duration of 150 μs. This stark contrast highlights the significant impact of varying EDM settings on the resulting surface characteristics, emphasizing the importance of careful parameter selection in achieving the desired surface finish in practical applications.

In a series of targeted trials conducted with a low discharge current of 1 A, researchers examined the effects of varying pulse-on times of 60, 150, and 200 μs. The findings revealed that there was no significant material removal across these trials. Specifically, Trials 2 through 4 demonstrated only minimal or negligible surface alterations. This lack of material removal can primarily be attributed to the insufficient energy generated during the process. The combination of low amperage and extended pulse-on durations limited the effectiveness of the treatment, as the energy input was not adequate to instigate meaningful discharges. Furthermore, the fixed pulse-off time of 20 μs contributed to this limitation by significantly reducing the frequency and intensity of the spark discharges. As a result of these conditions, the samples from these trials were classified as untreated, leading to the decision not to conduct any biological evaluations on them, as there were no notable changes to assess. This underlines the importance of optimizing both current settings and pulse durations in future experiments to achieve desired material modifications.

The microstructural characteristics of the samples processed through EDM are comprehensively illustrated in Fig. 5.4. In Fig. 5.4a, the surface morphology corresponding to a current of 10 A with an on-time of 60 μs (Trial 10) reveals minimal surface undulations. This observation indicates a notably smooth texture, with the lowest recorded roughness value of Ra = 0.42 μm. This exceptional surface quality can be attributed to the optimal coordination between the frequency of the spark

Table 5.2 Experimental array and surface roughness response

Trial No.	I (A)	P_{on} (μs)	Ra (μm)
1	1	20	1.15
2	1	60	0.48
3	1	150	0.49
4	1	200	0.48
5	5	20	1.23
6	5	60	1.21
7	5	150	0.89
8	5	200	1.40
9	10	20	1.31
10	10	60	0.42
11	10	150	0.49
12	10	200	1.16
13	16	20	1.06
14	16	60	2.39
15	16	150	2.47
16	16	200	1.42

Reproduced with permission from Taylor & Francis [5]

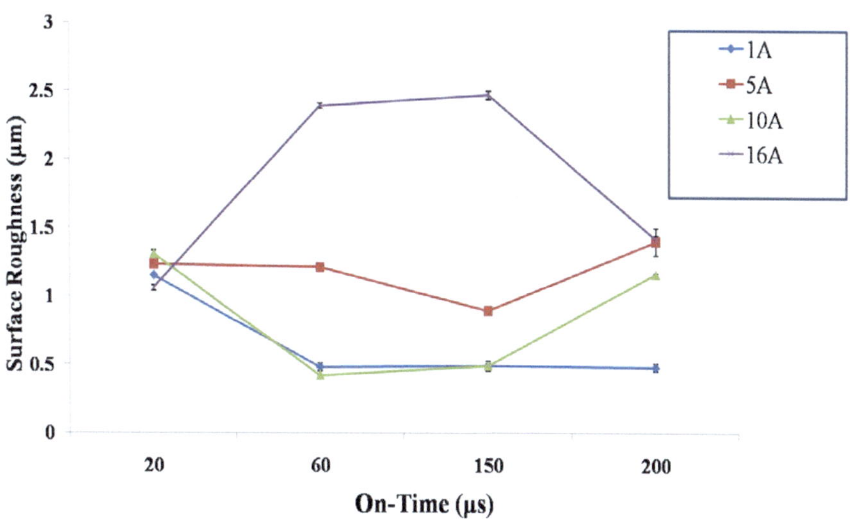

Fig. 5.3 EDM process parameter effect on surface roughness. Reproduced with permission from Taylor & Francis [5]

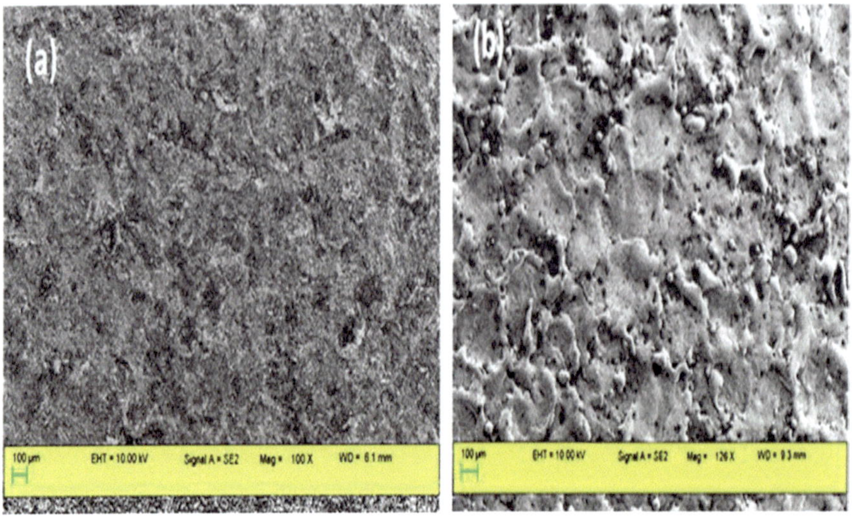

Fig. 5.4 Morphology of the machined surface obtained at different sets of parameters **a** $I = 10$ A; $P_{\text{on}} = 60$ μs; **b** $I = 16$ A; $P_{\text{on}} = 60$ μs. Reproduced with permission from Taylor & Francis [5]

energy and the efficiency of the debris flushing mechanism. This synergy allowed for the rapid removal of eroded particles from the machining zone, thus preventing the accumulation of debris that could impact surface finish. In contrast, when the current was increased to 16 A during Trial 14, as illustrated in Fig. 5.4b, the higher discharge energy produced a more complex surface topography. The pronounced ridges formed around the craters suggest a rougher surface texture, leading to increased irregularities and variations across the machined area. This difference in surface morphology highlights the critical relationship between electrical parameters during EDM processing and the resultant characteristics of the finished surface. The transition from a smooth to an uneven surface underscores the importance of optimizing machining conditions to achieve the desired surface quality in EDM applications.

The analysis revealed that the micro-roughness, which refers to the fine surface finishing observed in the samples, did not have a direct impact on their biological performance. This finding suggests that the subtle texture on a microscopic level may not significantly influence how the materials interact with biological systems. In contrast, the macro-roughness, which is characterized by its visibility to the naked eye, played a crucial role in fostering suitable conditions for interaction with surrounding tissues. This larger-scale roughness could enhance the material's ability to promote cellular adhesion and integration, thereby improving its overall biocompatibility and effectiveness in medical applications [6].

5.2.2 *In-Vitro Biocompatibility Test*

To thoroughly investigate the interaction between surfaces treated by electrical discharge machining (EDMed) and biological components such as tissue cells and human blood, we performed in-vitro cytotoxicity and hemolysis assays. These tests are crucial for understanding the biological response to materials used in biomedical applications. In the cytotoxicity assays, the test samples were exposed to two types of human cell lines: MCF-7 (Michigan Cancer Foundation-7) cells, which are derived from breast cancer tissue and are commonly used as a model for studying cancer biology, and HeLa cells, which originate from cervical carcinoma and serve as an important tool in cancer and genetics research. By analyzing the impact of the EDMed surfaces on these cell lines, we aimed to determine whether the materials exhibit cytotoxic properties that could inhibit cell growth or induce cell death. In the hemolysis assays, we evaluated the effect of the EDMed surfaces on human erythrocytes to assess the extent of RBC lysis. This is important because hemolysis can indicate potential adverse reactions when materials come into contact with blood in medical applications. By measuring the degree of RBC lysis, we can better understand how these surfaces interact with the blood and the implications for their use in biomedical implants or devices [7]. Overall, this comprehensive approach aims to provide insight into the biocompatibility of EDMed surfaces, which is essential for ensuring the safety and effectiveness of biomedical materials in clinical settings.

Effect of the EDM-Treated Samples on Hemolysis

The hemolytic activity of various samples is illustrated in Fig. 5.5, which provides a comprehensive comparison of the results. The positive control, Triton X™-100, resulted in complete hemolysis, achieving a 100% lysis rate of red blood cells, indicating its strong ability to disrupt cellular membranes. In contrast, the negative control, isotonic PBS at pH 7.4, showed a significantly lower hemolytic response, with only $4.53 \pm 2.61\%$ of the cells undergoing hemolysis. This minimal response demonstrates that PBS, as a physiologically balanced solution, effectively maintains cell integrity and highlights the potency of Triton X™-100 as an effective hemolytic agent.

In the study assessing hemolysis rates among various samples, the untreated group exhibited a notably elevated hemolysis rate in comparison to the negative control group, with a statistically significant difference ($p < 0.001$). Particularly alarming was Sample 6, which demonstrated a hemolysis rate of $30.86 \pm 4.97\%$. This high percentage indicates substantial damage to erythrocytes, raising concerns about the sample's biocompatibility. Furthermore, Samples 1, 5, 7, 10, 13, and 15 each displayed a statistically significant increase in hemolysis rates when compared to the negative control, with p-values below 0.05. This suggests that these samples may also have adverse effects on red blood cells, warranting further investigation into their safety for potential applications. Conversely, Samples 8, 9, 11, 12, 14, and 16 did not show any statistically significant differences in hemolysis levels relative

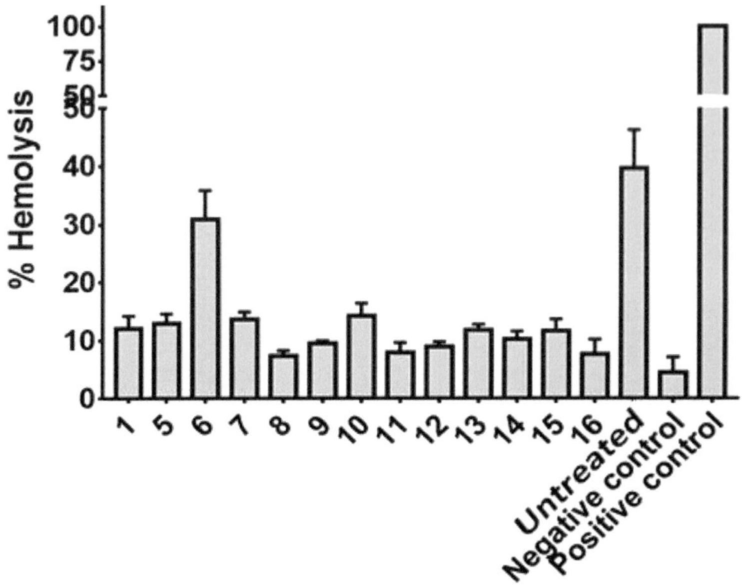

Fig. 5.5 Percentage hemolysis of EDM-treated samples. All values expressed as mean ± SD, at $n = 3$. Reproduced with permission from Taylor & Francis [5]

to the negative control ($p > 0.05$). This finding implies that these samples have benefitted from surface modifications that enhance their hemocompatibility, making them potentially safer for biomedical use. Overall, the results underscore the importance of evaluating hemolytic activity in assessing the safety and efficacy of materials intended for contact with blood.

The findings were further substantiated through a detailed analysis using SEM to examine the morphology of RBCs, as illustrated in Fig. 5.6. The SEM images revealed that RBCs exposed to Samples 1, 5, 7, 10, 13, and 15 exhibited significant signs of aggregation, deformation, and clumping. These morphological changes suggest that the cells experienced considerable cellular stress or damage, likely due to adverse interactions with the tested samples. In contrast, RBCs that interacted with Samples 8, 9, 11, 12, 14, and 16 maintained a morphology consistent with that of the negative control group, indicating that these samples did not induce any noticeable harm or stress to the cells. Their appearance was characterized by intact cell membranes and uniform shapes, which are typical of healthy RBCs. Additionally, the SEM images from Samples 1, 5, 7, 10, 13, and 15 displayed blurry backgrounds, which likely indicate the presence of protein agglomeration on the surfaces of the RBCs. This phenomenon suggests that protein interactions may be contributing to the observed cellular abnormalities. In contrast, the backgrounds of the images for the remaining samples and the negative control group were relatively clear, pointing to minimal or absent protein deposition on the RBC surfaces. This distinction further highlights the differences in cellular responses to varying test samples and underscores the importance of careful assessment in evaluating the biocompatibility of these materials.

Sample 8 demonstrated a significantly lower percentage of hemolysis when compared to its untreated counterparts. This finding suggests that Sample 8 has enhanced hemocompatibility, which is crucial for applications involving blood contact. The observed reduction in hemolysis aligns with the overall improvement in blood compatibility noted in the EDM-treated samples, highlighting the effectiveness of this treatment method. Despite the promising results, it is important to acknowledge that not all treatment parameters yielded optimal hemolysis reduction. Nevertheless, the study successfully identified several key modifications that contribute to improved hemocompatibility. These modifications could serve as a foundation for future research aimed at further enhancing the safety and effectiveness of biomedical materials in blood-contacting applications.

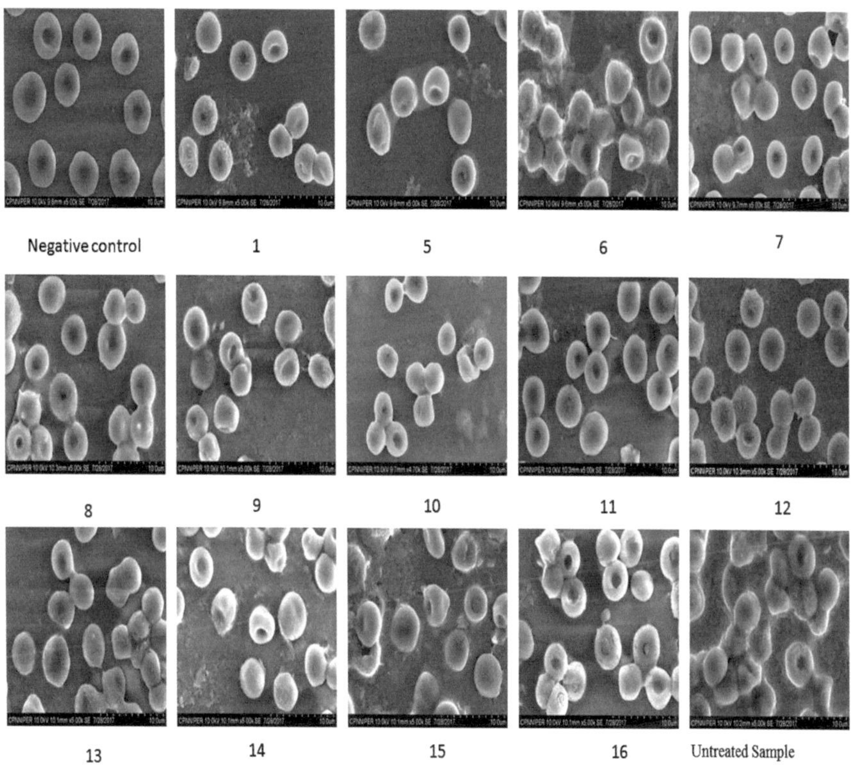

Fig. 5.6 Comparative images of RBC morphology of different samples (samples from Trial 2, Trial 3, and Trial 4 are represented as untreated surfaces). Reproduced with permission from Taylor & Francis [5]

Effect of the EDM-Treated Samples on Cytocompatibility

The cytocompatibility of both EDM-treated and untreated samples was evaluated by calculating the percentage of cellular viability, as illustrated in Figs. 5.7 and 5.8. For this assessment, we utilized the MCF-7 and HeLa cell lines, which are commonly used models for studying cancer cell behavior. The results revealed that the Cr–Co alloy specimens exhibited a significant reduction in cell viability when compared to the negative control group, which consisted of cells cultured on a standard coverslip. This decrease in viability indicates that the Cr–Co alloy may have cytotoxic effects on these cell lines. Interestingly, the EDM-treated samples numbered 5, 12, and 15 demonstrated no significant difference in cell viability relative to the positive control group, which included untreated Cr–Co samples. This finding suggests that the EDM treatment may enhance the biocompatibility of the Cr–Co alloy, allowing it to maintain cellular viability at levels comparable to untreated samples. Overall, these results provide valuable insight into the potential applications of Cr–Co alloys in biomedical settings, particularly in the context of implants or devices used in close contact with living tissues.

Among the specimens treated with EDM, a noteworthy observation was made in Samples 1, 6, 7, 8, 9, 10, 11, 13, 14, and 16, which exhibited enhanced cell viability compared to the positive control. Specifically, these samples showed viability values ranging from 39 to 54%. Among them, Sample 8 stood out, achieving an impressive cell viability of approximately 80% when compared to the control group. In greater detail, the analysis revealed that the viability of MCF-7 (breast cancer) and HeLa (cervical cancer) cells exposed to Sample 8 was found to be 2.05 and 2.43 times greater than that of the untreated specimens, respectively. This significant increase

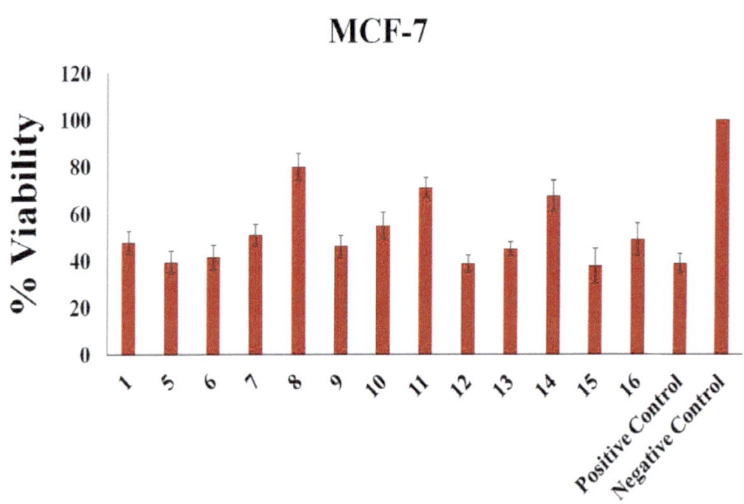

Fig. 5.7 Percentage viability of MCF-7 cells upon different samples. Reproduced with permission from Taylor & Francis [5]

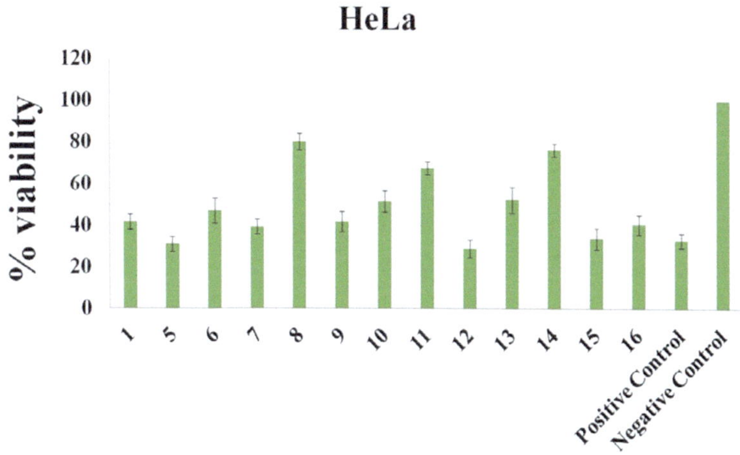

Fig. 5.8 Percentage viability of HeLa cells upon different samples

underscores the potential effectiveness of the EDM treatment in promoting cell health and resilience. Conversely, it is important to note that Samples 12 and 15 exhibited viability levels nearly identical to those of the untreated control, suggesting that these specific treatments did not confer the same positive effects as those seen in the other samples. The consistency of these findings was further supported by the results of in-vitro hemocompatibility assays, which assessed the interaction between the treated materials and blood components. These assays confirmed a favorable biological response, indicating a positive blood–material interaction. Overall, the results strongly suggest that the EDM-modified surfaces exhibit not only enhanced biocompatibility but also improved safety profiles [8, 9]. This highlights their promising potential for application in orthopedic implants, where material compatibility with biological tissues is crucial for successful integration and long-term functionality.

5.2.3 XRD Analysis

Figure 5.9 presents a detailed comparison of the X-ray diffraction (XRD) patterns obtained from two different surfaces: the untreated surface and the surface that has been modified through EDM. The XRD patterns provide critical insights into the crystallographic structures and phase compositions of both surfaces, highlighting how EDM alters the material characteristics. By analyzing the differences in peak intensity and positions, we can better understand the effects of EDM on the surface properties, such as stress, texture, and possible phase transformation, as compared to the untreated state.

All the examined specimens were composed of essential compounds containing chromium (Cr), iron (Fe), molybdenum (Mo), and cobalt (Co). The specific phases

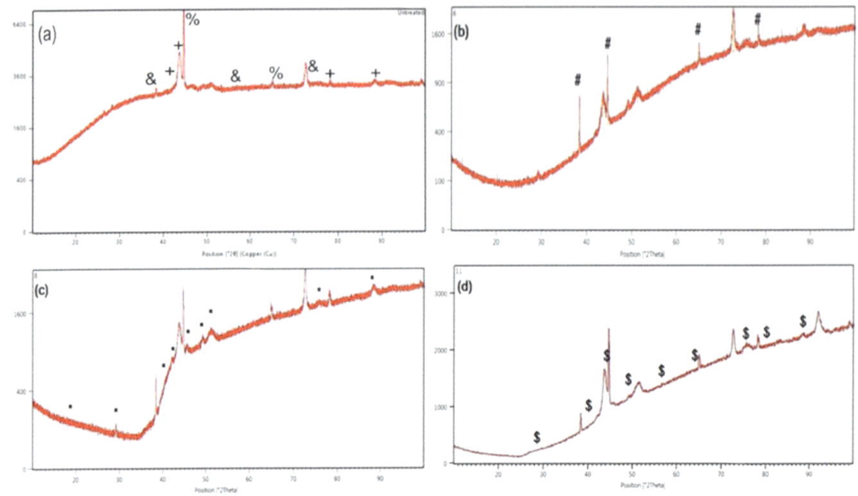

Fig. 5.9 XRD pattern of Co–Cr specimen **a** untreated surface (mark (plus): + corresponds to phases of cobalt; mark (percentage): % corresponds to phases of chromium; mark (and): & corresponds to phases of molybdenum); **b** Trial 6: EDMed surface (mark (hash): # corresponds to carbides phase); **c** Trial 8: EDMed surface (mark (star): * corresponds to phosphide phase); **d** Trial 11: EDMed surface (mark (dollar): $ corresponds to oxide phase). Reproduced with permission from Taylor & Francis [5]

identified included $CoFe_3$, $CrSi_2$, and $Co_{3.31}Mo_{3.31}Mn_{3.31}$, which are known for their unique properties and applications in various industrial contexts. After undergoing surface modification through EDM utilizing varying spark energies, several distinct phases were observed. Notably, a tetragonal phosphide phase ($Cr_{2.4}Ni_{0.6}P_1$) emerged, along with cubic phases of carbides and oxides, particularly Cr_3O. This phase of development is significant as it suggests alterations in the material's electronic and corrosion-resistant properties due to EDM [10, 11]. The morphological and chemical changes induced by EDM were found to positively impact cellular compatibility, which is crucial for applications in biomedicine and tissue engineering. The processes involved in EDM not only modified the surface structure but also enhanced biocompatibility by facilitating the formation of phosphide and oxide layers. These layers acted as favorable substrates that improved cellular attachment and proliferation. The creation of an oxide film was particularly important, as it provided a protective barrier against intergranular corrosion, a common challenge in metallic materials exposed to harsh environments. This oxide layer significantly contributes to the material's longevity and performance in biomedical applications [12]. These transformative surface phase changes became especially evident when the applied EDM spark energy was varied between 960 and 1500 J, which is illustrated in Fig. 5.10. The range of energy used plays a critical role in determining the extent and nature of the phase transformations observed, emphasizing the importance of precise control over processing parameters in the EDM technique.

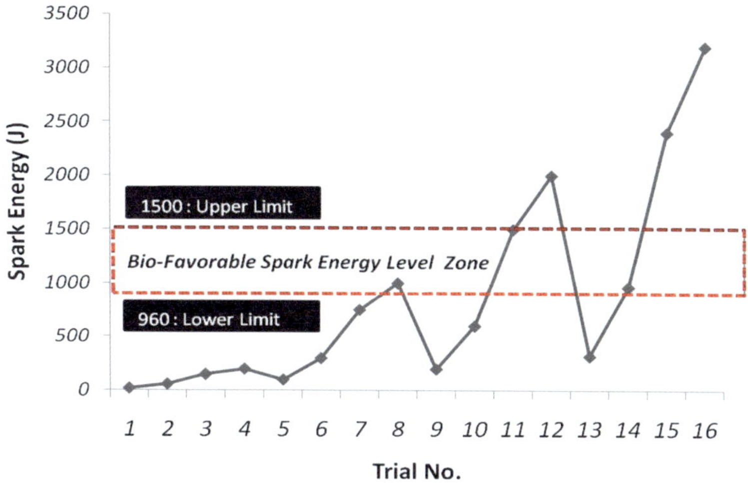

Fig. 5.10 Illustration of spark energy versus trials and bio-favorable spark energy zone. Reproduced with permission from Taylor & Francis [5]

The study focused on the surface morphology and elemental composition of the most biologically compatible sample from our trials (Trial 8), utilizing advanced techniques such as SEM and energy dispersive X-ray spectroscopy (EDX) for a comprehensive analysis. As illustrated in Fig. 5.11, the machined surface, subjected to an energy application of 1000 J, displayed intricate surface features marked by micro-porosity in the range of approximately 3–5 μm [13, 14]. This micro-porosity, alongside the presence of resolidified molten droplets, contributes significantly to the surface's ability to facilitate cell attachment and promote cellular proliferation, key factors for successful biological integration [15, 16]. Furthermore, the EDX analysis revealed the presence of phosphide compounds on the treated surface. These compounds are hypothesized to play a crucial role in enhancing the bioactivity of the material by improving its interaction with biological systems [17, 18]. Overall, the combination of these morphological characteristics and chemical enhancements suggests that the surface treatment applied to Trial 8 effectively improves the material's compatibility for biomedical applications.

5.3 Conclusions

The surface characteristics and biological responses of cobalt-chromium (Co–Cr) alloy knee joint specimens were thoroughly evaluated following treatment with EDM. This advanced machining technique employs high-voltage electrical discharges to precisely remove material and modify surface properties. During the investigation, we found that applying spark energies within the range of 960–1500 J significantly

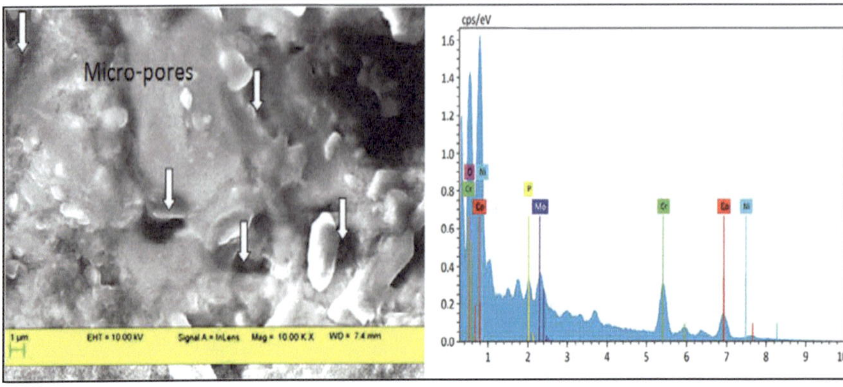

Fig. 5.11 Combined SEM images and EDX-ray spectra of EDMed surface of Trial 8 ($I = 5$ A; $P_{on} = 200$ μs; micropores are indicated with arrows). Reproduced with permission from Taylor & Francis [5]

influenced the surface's physical structure. This process resulted in the creation of macro-scale surface roughness, which can enhance mechanical interlocking with biological tissues, as well as the formation of micro-scale features such as micropores and redeposited molten droplets. This combination of textures is crucial as it fosters a more favorable environment for cellular adhesion, viability, and proliferation when compared to untreated specimens, highlighting the potential of this specific spark energy range to improve biological compatibility. To further assess the hemocompatibility of the EDM-treated surfaces, we conducted in-vitro hemolysis tests. These tests demonstrated that the modified surfaces exhibited significantly better interaction with blood components, indicating lower rates of hemolysis and thus enhanced compatibility with biological fluids. Particularly noteworthy was the sample processed under conditions of a 5 A discharge current and a pulse duration of 200 μs (Trial 8). This specific treatment not only enhanced the surface's physical characteristics but also led to the formation of phosphide phases. These phases have been associated with improved biocompatibility and hemocompatibility, suggesting that they play a beneficial role in preventing adverse reactions in the human body. Overall, the EDM technique effectively merges the processes of material removal and surface modification. This dual approach not only achieves enhanced dimensional accuracy but also holds significant promise for improving clinical outcomes in orthopedic applications. The findings suggest that EDM-treated Co–Cr alloy knee joint specimens have the potential to provide better integration and performance within the biological environment of the body.

References

1. Mahajan A, Sidhu SS (2019) In vitro corrosion and hemocompatibility evaluation of electrical discharge treated cobalt–chromium implant. J Mater Res 34(8):1363–1370
2. Dora CP, Kushwah V, Katiyar SS, Kumar P, Pillay V, Suresh S, Jain S (2017) Improved metabolic stability and therapeutic efficacy of a novel molecular gemcitabine phospholipid complex. Int J Pharm 530(1–2):113–127
3. Longster GH, Buckley T, Sikorski J, Tovey LA (1972) Scanning electron microscope studies of red cell morphology. Vox Sang 22(2):161–170
4. Srivastava V, Negi AS, Kumar JK, Gupta MM, Khanuja SP (2005) Plant-based anticancer molecules: a chemical and biological profile of some important leads. Bioorg Med Chem 13(21):5892–5908
5. Mahajan A, Sidhu SS (2018) Enhancing biocompatibility of Co–Cr alloy implants via electrical discharge process. Mater Technol 33(8):524–531
6. Horwitz SB, Chang CK, Grollman AP (1971) Studies on camptothecin: I. Effects on nucleic acid and protein synthesis. Mol Pharmacol 7(6):632–644
7. Ahmadian S, Barar J, Saei AA, Fakhree MAA, Omidi Y (2009) Cellular toxicity of nanogenomedicine in MCF-7 cell line: MTT assay. J Vis Exp 26:1191
8. Harcuba P, Bacakova L, Strasky J, Bacakova M, Novotna K, Janecek M (2012) Surface treatment by electric discharge machining of Ti–6Al–4V alloy for potential application in orthopaedics. J Mech Behav Biomed Mater 7:96–105
9. Lee BE, Ho S, Mestres G, Ott MK, Koshy P, Grandfield K (2016) Dual-topography electrical discharge machining of titanium to improve biocompatibility. Surf Coat Technol 296:149–156
10. Singh G, Ablyaz TR, Shlykov ES, Muratov KR, Bhui AS, Sidhu SS (2020) Enhancing corrosion and wear resistance of Ti6Al4V alloy using CNTs mixed electro-discharge process. Micromachines 11(9):850
11. Al-Amin M, Abdul-Rani AM, Danish M, Rubaiee S, Mahfouz AB, Thompson HM et al (2021) Investigation of coatings, corrosion and wear characteristics of machined biomaterials through hydroxyapatite mixed-EDM process: a review. Materials 14(13):3597
12. Jenko M, Gorensek M, Godec M, Hodnik M, Batic BS, Donik C, Grant JT, Dolinar D (2018) Surface chemistry and microstructure of metallic biomaterials for hip and knee endoprostheses. Appl Surf Sci 427:584–593
13. Li G, Wang L, Pan W, Yang F, Jiang W, Wu X, Kong X, Dai K, Hao Y (2016) In vitro and in vivo study of additive manufactured porous Ti6Al4V scaffolds for repairing bone defects. Sci Rep 6:34072
14. Gittens RA, McLachlan T, Olivares-Navarrete R, Cai Y, Berner S, Tannenbaum R, Boyan BD (2011) The effects of combined micron-/submicron-scale surface roughness and nanoscale features on cell proliferation and differentiation. Biomaterials 32(13):3395–3403
15. Mahajan A, Devgan S, Sidhu SS (2021) Surface alteration of biomedical alloys by electrical discharge treatment for enhancing the electrochemical corrosion, tribological and biological performances. Surf Coat Technol 405:126583
16. Devgan S, Mahajan A, Sidhu SS (2021) Multi-walled carbon nanotubes in powder mixed electrical discharge machining: an experimental study, state of the art and feasibility prospect. Appl Phys A 127(11):806
17. Al-Amin M, Abdul-Rani AM, Rao TVVLN, Danish M, Rubaiee S, bin Mahfouz A, Wani MF (2022) Investigation of machining and modified surface features of 316L steel through novel hybrid of HA/CNT added-EDM process. Mater Chem Phys 276:125320
18. Singh G, Sidhu SS, Bains PS, Singh M, Bhui AS (2020) On surface modification of Ti alloy by electro discharge coating using hydroxyapatite powder mixed dielectric with graphite tool. J Bio Tribo-Corros 6(3):91

Chapter 6
In-Vitro Corrosion Investigation of Co–Cr Alloy (Stage II)

This chapter provides a comprehensive analysis of the behavior of medical-grade cobalt-chromium (Co–Cr) alloy when subjected to electrical discharge treatment. We investigate how different spark energy levels influence the alloy's properties and performance, as well as the effects of various dielectric media used during the treatment process. By systematically varying the spark energy and exploring a range of dielectric environments, we aim to understand the implications of these parameters on the microstructural changes, surface characteristics, and overall functional behavior of the Co–Cr alloy. This research is crucial for optimizing the alloy's application in medical devices, where performance and biocompatibility are of paramount importance.

6.1 Description of Stage II Experimentation

The Stage II experimentation delves into the in-vitro corrosion analysis of medical-grade cobalt-chromium (Co–Cr) alloy surfaces, specifically focusing on those modified through electrical discharge treatment (EDT). This process was conducted at various energy levels to assess how alterations in treatment parameters impact the corrosion resistance of the alloys. The energy levels during treatment were precisely regulated by modifying specific parameters, including the intensity of the electric current, the duration of the pulse-on phase, and the length of the pulse-off intervals, all of which are elaborated upon in the design of experiments. To facilitate the treatment, three distinct types of electrode materials were utilized: graphite (C), tungsten (W), and copper-tungsten (Cu–W). Each material contributes unique characteristics to the electrical discharge process, influencing the modification of the Co–Cr alloy surfaces. These treatments were performed in two different dielectric environments, mineral oil and deionized water, each chosen for its distinct properties that may affect the discharge treatment efficacy and subsequent corrosion resistance.

© The Author(s), under exclusive license to Springer Nature Singapore Pte Ltd. 2026

A. Mahajan et al., *Surface Modification of Co–Cr Alloy for Orthopaedic Applications*, Biomedical Materials for Multi-functional Applications,
https://doi.org/10.1007/978-981-95-4029-7_6

Following the surface modifications, a series of electrochemical potentiodynamic polarization tests were conducted to rigorously evaluate the corrosion resistance of both the untreated and treated alloy surfaces. These tests allowed for a detailed analysis of the electrochemical behavior of the surfaces in simulated physiological environments. Furthermore, in-vitro assessments of hemocompatibility were carried out on the samples that exhibited enhanced corrosion resistance. This involved an examination of red blood cell lysis, a critical measure of compatibility with human blood, providing insights into how the modified surfaces might interact with biological systems. Through this multifaceted approach, the research aims to establish a comprehensive understanding of the relationship between electrical discharge treatment and the corrosion resistance and biocompatibility of Co–Cr alloys in medical applications.

6.1.1 Electrochemical Corrosion Measurements

To evaluate the electrochemical corrosion behavior of Co–Cr alloys, a series of potentiodynamic polarization tests was conducted on both untreated and EDM-processed samples. These tests were carried out using a potentiostat/galvanostat system, manufactured by Autolab in the Netherlands, which was integrated with Nova software to facilitate data acquisition and analysis. Detailed specifications of the electrochemical setup, including device parameters and configurations, can be found in Table 6.1. A simulated body fluid (SBF) environment was used to better replicate physiological conditions, utilizing Ringer's solution sourced from Nice Chemical Pvt. Ltd. in Cochin, India. The solution's pH was maintained at 7.2 to closely mimic the conditions found in human bodily fluids. The precise chemical formulation of the solution included 9 g/L of NaCl, 0.43 g/L of KCl, 0.2 g/L of $NaHCO_3$, and 0.24 g/L of $CaCl_2$, ensuring adequate ionic balance for corrosion testing. Prior to conducting the corrosion tests, all Co–Cr samples were immersed in the SBF for a duration of 24 h. This soaking period allowed the samples to reach a state of equilibrium and stabilization with the test environment, which is crucial for accurate readings during polarization. In each test, the Co–Cr alloy specimen acted as the working electrode, while a platinum (Pt) rod was employed as the counter electrode, and a saturated Ag/AgCl calomel electrode served as the reference electrode. To ensure a consistent and controlled data set, a scan rate of 1 mV/s was maintained throughout the experiments. Furthermore, to uphold the integrity of the results, fresh Ringer's solution was prepared for each trial, minimizing the potential for contamination or interference. To enhance the reliability and replicability of findings, each set of tests was performed three times under identical conditions, allowing for a robust statistical analysis of the corrosion behavior exhibited by the Co–Cr alloys. This comprehensive approach aims to provide insights that are crucial for determining the suitability of these materials in biomedical applications.

The evaluation of the corrosion rate, current density, and corrosion potential was conducted using Tafel extrapolation plots, which are essential tools for

Table 6.1 Specification of electrochemical unit

Electrochemical unit	Description
Potentiostat/galvanostat	• Maximum current ± 2 A • Compliance voltage ± 30 V • Potential range ± 10 V • Potential resolution 0.3 μV • Potentiostat bandwidth 1 MHz
Reference electrode	• Saturated calomel electrode • Non-aqueous Ag/Ag^+ reference electrode • Hg/HgO reference electrode • Mercury/mercurous sulfate electrode • Ag/AgCl reference electrode
Working electrode	• Glassy carbon working electrode • Metal electrode • Platinum working electrode • Gold working electrode
Counter electrode	• Platinum conductivity/plate/wire/mesh electrode • Graphite rod/electrode
Control software	NOVA

Reproduced with permission from Springer Nature [1]

analyzing electrochemical reactions. To obtain accurate polarization measurements, we conducted tests within a potential range of − 0.1 to + 0.1 mV with respect to the open circuit potential, allowing for a comprehensive assessment of the electrochemical behavior of the material. The complete electrochemical setup, which includes all necessary components and configurations for these measurements, is illustrated in Fig. 6.1. To quantify the corrosion rate, we employed Eq. 6.1 [2], which allows us to express the rate of corrosion in mm/year. This detailed approach enables a clearer understanding of the material's performance in corrosive environments.

$$\text{C.R.} = \frac{I_{\text{corr}} * K * \text{EW}}{d * A} \tag{6.1}$$

where

C.R. Corrosion rate (mm/year)
I_{corr} Corrosion current in amperes, where 1 nA = 10^{-9} A
K Constant, value = 3272 mm/(A cm year)
EW Equivalent weight of Co–Cr alloy, value = 28.011 g/mol
d Density of alloy value 8.3 g/cm^3
A Area of substrate.

The analysis of variance (ANOVA) was utilized to thoroughly evaluate the corrosion behavior of the treated substrates. This statistical method allows us to determine how various factors contribute to corrosion rates. Specifically, a higher F-test value associated with a particular factor indicates a more significant impact on controlling

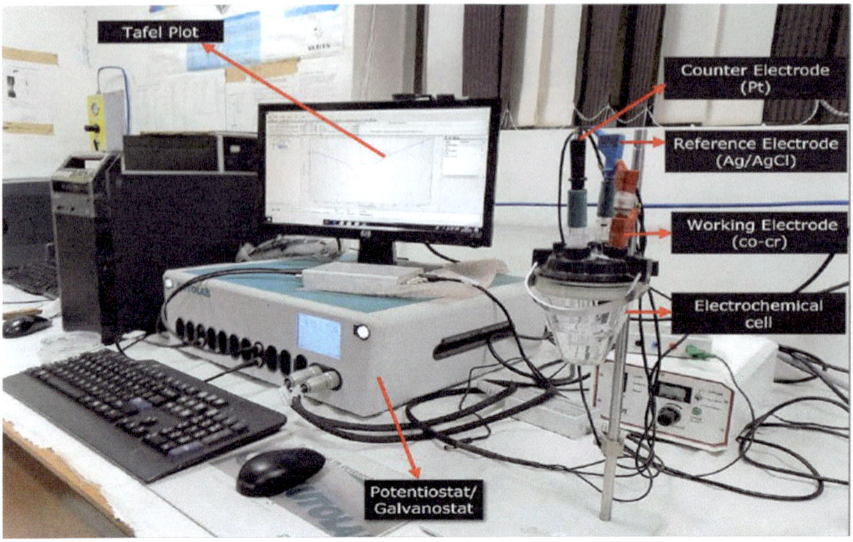

Fig. 6.1 Experimental setup of the electrochemical workstation. Reproduced with permission from Springer Nature [1]

the corrosion rate. In addition to the *F*-test, the *p*-value is employed to assess the statistical significance of each parameter; a lower *p*-value suggests that the factor has a meaningful effect on corrosion behavior. At this stage of the analysis, we focused on examining several key corrosion characteristics, which include:

Response name:	Corrosion rate
Response type:	Lower the better criteria (S/N ratio)
Units:	mm/year.

6.1.2 *In-Vitro Hemolysis Test*

The hemolysis test was conducted to evaluate the compatibility of surfaces treated through electrical discharge with human blood, with particular emphasis on those demonstrating high corrosion resistance. When it comes to medical implants, the potential for metal ions to be released into the bloodstream poses a significant risk, as these ions can interact negatively with blood components or surrounding tissues, ultimately leading to detrimental effects on patient health. To mitigate these risks, samples that exhibited superior corrosion resistance were selected for detailed analysis to assess their hemocompatibility, or their ability to coexist with blood without causing harmful reactions. The hemolysis test was executed according to the established procedures outlined in Stage I, which included specific incubation times and conditions to ensure reliable results. After the incubation period, the 24-well plates used for the hemolysis test were visually assessed, as illustrated in Fig. 6.2. This

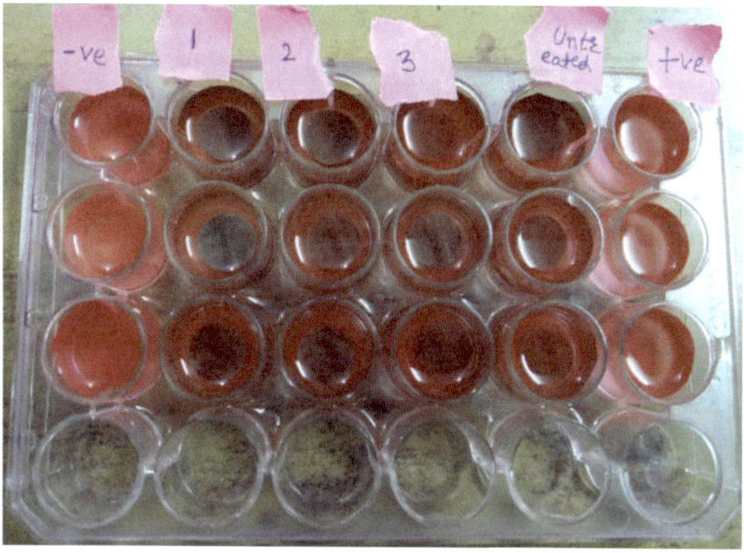

Fig. 6.2 Pictorial view of the well plate and immersed sample for the hemolysis test

figure provides a comprehensive view of the test setup, allowing for a clearer understanding of the experimental process. Additionally, the morphology of the RBCs was examined under a CX41 Olympus microscope, sourced from P. Bhogilal Pvt. Ltd. in India. The examination focused on identifying any alterations to the RBCs that may indicate hemolytic activity, allowing for a thorough evaluation of the compatibility of the treated surfaces with human blood.

6.2 Results and Discussion

This study presents a comprehensive examination of an experiment conducted on Co–Cr biomedical alloy samples, which are widely used in medical applications due to their excellent mechanical properties and biocompatibility. The experiment employed three distinct types of tool electrodes to evaluate their effects on the alloy's performance: a fine-grained graphite electrode, characterized by a particle size of approximately 5 μm; a tungsten electrode, known for its durability and conductivity; and a tungsten-copper composite electrode, which combines the advantageous properties of both materials. The primary objective of this research was to investigate the corrosion resistance and hemocompatibility of the Co–Cr alloy substrates that were treated with these electrodes. Corrosion resistance is vital for the longevity and safety of biomedical implants, while hemocompatibility is crucial for ensuring that materials do not trigger adverse reactions when in contact with blood. By comparing the performance of the alloy samples treated with each electrode, this study aims to provide valuable insights into optimizing the selection of materials for biomedical applications, ultimately contributing to improved patient outcomes.

The experimental procedure was designed based on an L18 orthogonal array, which allows for a systematic evaluation of multiple variables simultaneously. This design included five key independent parameters: the electric current applied, the duration of the pulse-on time, the duration of the pulse-off time, the type of electrode material used, and the choice of dielectric fluid. Each of these factors was selected to understand their influence on the corrosion rates observed during the experiment. The experimental setup was carefully arranged to ensure consistent results, and the corrosion rates were calculated using Eq. 6.1, which quantifies the rate of material degradation. The findings, including the specific conditions under which each measurement was taken and the corresponding corrosion rates, are detailed in Table 6.2. This table serves as a comprehensive reference for understanding how variations in independent parameters affect corrosion behavior.

Table 6.2 L18 experimental design layout and results

Trial No.	I (A)	P_{on} (μs)	P_{off} (μs)	Electrode	Dielectric medium	Corrosion rate (mm/year) (Avg. ± S.D.)
1	5	60	60	Gr	EDM oil	0.002961 ± 0.0003
2	5	150	150	W	EDM oil	0.039954 ± 0.01
3	5	200	200	W–Cu	EDM oil	0.030189 ± 0.005
4	10	60	60	W	EDM oil	0.021432 ± 0.006
5	10	150	150	W–Cu	EDM oil	0.000581 ± 0.0002
6	10	200	200	Gr	EDM oil	0.005607 ± 0.001
7	16	60	150	Gr	EDM oil	0.018208 ± 0.006
8	16	150	200	W	EDM oil	0.060112 ± 0.02
9	16	200	60	W–Cu	EDM oil	0.00108 ± 0.003
10	5	60	200	W–Cu	Deionized water	0.015751 ± 0.005
11	5	150	60	Gr	Deionized water	0.024358 ± 0.02
12	5	200	150	W	Deionized water	0.019277 ± 0.03
13	10	60	150	W–Cu	Deionized water	0.000388 ± 0.0002
14	10	150	200	Gr	Deionized water	0.02065 ± 0.005
15	10	200	60	W	Deionized water	0.013052 ± 0.006
16	16	60	200	W	Deionized water	0.019941 ± 0.03
17	16	150	60	W–Cu	Deionized water	0.012539 ± 0.002
18	16	200	150	Gr	Deionized water	0.004305 ± 0.003

Reproduced with permission from Springer Nature [1]

6.2.1 Statistical Analysis

The corrosion characteristics of the materials were thoroughly evaluated, focusing on several key parameters: corrosion potential (E_{corr}), corrosion current density (I_{corr}), corrosion rate (C.R.), and polarization resistance (R_p). These parameters were determined by analyzing the intersection of cathodic and anodic Tafel slopes, utilizing the advanced capabilities of Nova computer software for precise data interpretation. To assess the effect of various factors on the corrosion rate (C.R.) of the machined surfaces, a statistical analysis known as analysis of variance (ANOVA) was performed. This analysis allowed for a comprehensive comparison of the corrosion rates across different sample conditions. The resulting data and insights from this analysis are presented in detail in the final column of Table 6.3, providing a clear overview of the corrosion behavior observed in the experiments conducted.

Factors that exhibit higher F-test values suggest a stronger influence on the corrosion rate, which is a critical metric in evaluating the longevity and durability of materials in various environments. Additionally, the p-value associated with each parameter provides insight into the statistical significance of its effect; a lower p-value indicates a more substantial influence. In this specific analysis, the electrode material was determined to be the most significant factor affecting corrosion resistance, with the order of influence continuing with pulse-on time and pulse-off time. Notably, the dielectric medium displayed minimal impact on the corrosion rate and was therefore excluded from further evaluations for clarity and focus in the analysis (refer to Table 6.3 for detailed insights). Figure 6.3 effectively illustrates the main effects of the input variables on corrosion resistance, highlighting the conditions under which optimal performance is achieved. Specifically, the analysis revealed that the best corrosion resistance was obtained when EDM was conducted using a tungsten-copper (W–Cu) composite electrode in deionized water. The ideal experimental parameters for achieving this optimal performance included a current of 10 A, a pulse-on time of 200 μs, and a pulse-off time set to the shortest duration of 60 μs.

Table 6.3 Analysis of variance for corrosion rate

Factors	Sum of squares	DOF	Variance	F-ratio	p-value (% contribution)
Current	0.000458	2	0.000229	2.34	0.158 (8.3%)
Pulse-on	0.000751	2	0.000376	3.84	0.068[b] (18.3%)
Pulse-off	0.000599	2	0.000300	3.07	0.10[b] (13.4%)
Electrode	0.001256	2	0.000628	6.42	0.022[a] (35.1%)
Dielectric medium[c]	0.000138	1	0.000138	1.41	0.269 (pooled)
Error	0.000782	8	0.000098	–	–

Reproduced with permission from Springer Nature [1]

[a] Most significant (95%)

[b] Significant (90%)

[c] Pooled factor

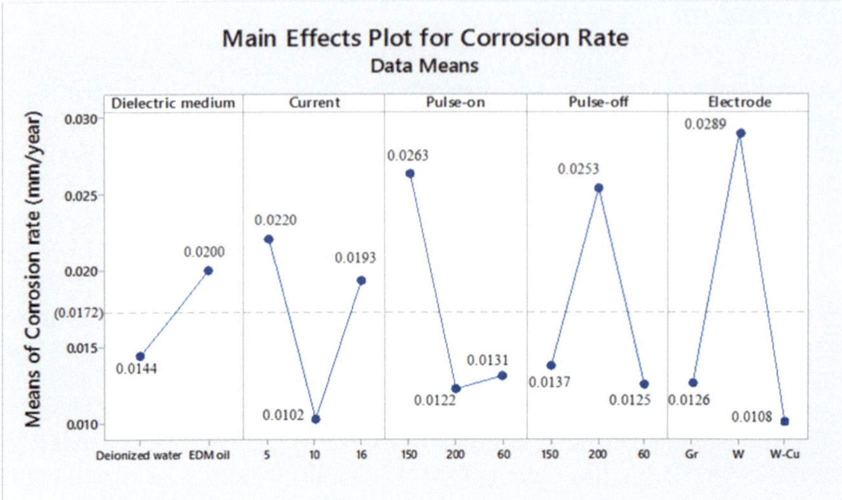

Fig. 6.3 Main effect plot for corrosion rate. Reproduced with permission from Springer Nature [1]

The results indicated that the W–Cu machined surface offered exceptional corrosion resistance, measuring just 0.0108 mm/year. In contrast, the surface machined with a tungsten electrode alone demonstrated a significantly lower resistance, with a measurement of 0.0289 mm/year. Among all the parameters analyzed, the variation introduced by changing the electrode material was the most pronounced, reinforcing the conclusion that the choice of electrode material is a critical determinant of corrosion resistance in electrical discharge machining applications. This insight can guide future research and practical applications aimed at enhancing material resilience in corrosive environments.

6.2.2 *Electrochemical Corrosion Analysis*

Figure 6.4 provides a detailed comparison of the potentiodynamic polarization curves for both untreated and selectively electrical discharge-treated cobalt-chromium (Co–Cr) samples. The untreated sample demonstrated a corrosion potential (E_{corr}) of −136.26 mV, indicating a relatively high susceptibility to corrosion in its environment. Additionally, it exhibited a corrosion current density (I_{corr}) of 181.26 nA/cm^2, which reflects the rate at which corrosion occurs. This untreated specimen also recorded a corrosion rate (C.R.) of 0.0020251 mm/year, a critical metric for assessing the material's longevity and durability in practical applications. The data highlights the effectiveness of electrical discharge treatment in enhancing the corrosion resistance of Co–Cr alloys, an important consideration in biomedical and industrial applications.

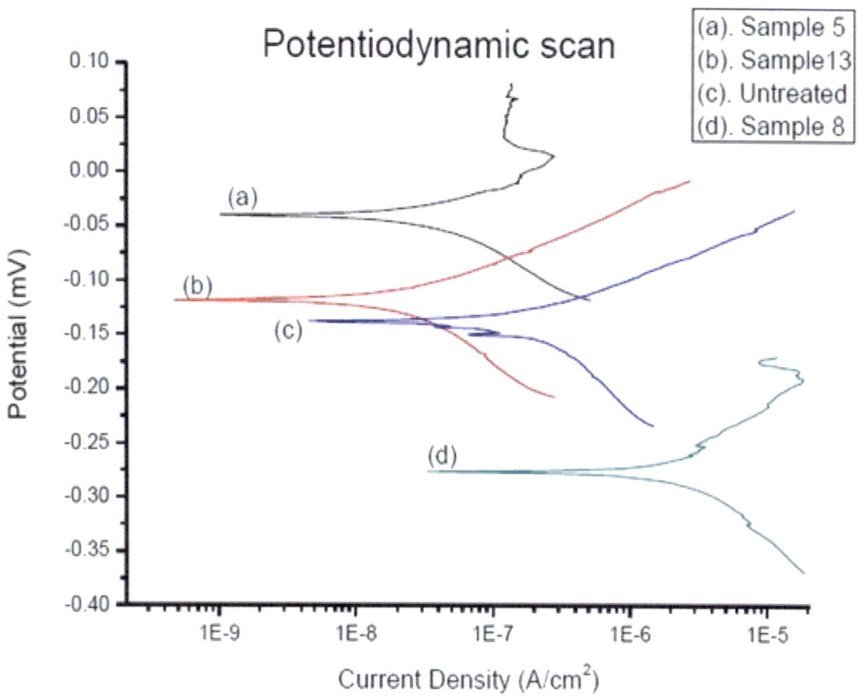

Fig. 6.4 Potentiodynamic polarization curves of **a** Sample 5 (I = 10 A, P_{on} = 150 μs, P_{off} = 150 μs, electrode = W–Cu, EDM oil), **b** Sample 13 (I = 10 A, P_{on} = 60 μs, P_{off} = 150 μs, electrode = W–Cu, deionized water), **c** untreated sample, **d** Sample 8 (I = 16 A, P_{on} = 150 μs, P_{off} = 200 μs, electrode = W, EDM oil). Reproduced with permission from Springer Nature [1]

The findings indicated that the sample processed during Trial 13 exhibited exceptional corrosion resistance, recording a corrosion rate of just 0.0003 mm/year. This impressive result highlights the effectiveness of the surface modification applied in this trial. In addition, samples from Trial 5, which recorded a corrosion rate of 0.0005 mm/year, and Trial 9, with a corrosion rate of 0.001 mm/year, also showed significantly reduced corrosion rates in comparison to the untreated specimen. These results collectively suggest that the surface treatments utilized in Trials 5 and 9 also contributed to enhanced corrosion resistance. Conversely, the sample treated under Trial 8 presented a concerning outcome, as it displayed a considerably higher corrosion rate, exceeding that of the untreated surface. This reversal in performance indicates a potential failure in the surface modification process or an adverse effect resulting from the specific treatment applied during Trial 8, suggesting a reduction in corrosion resistance instead of the expected improvement. The corrosion parameters, meticulously derived using the Tafel extrapolation method, are summarized in Table 6.4, which provides a clear comparison of the corrosion rates across the different trials. These findings underscore the critical importance of selecting appropriate surface modification techniques to optimize corrosion resistance in materials.

Figure 6.5a, d provide a detailed representation of the surface morphology of the EDM-treated samples. These images reveal an uneven texture, characterized by the presence of micro-pores and re-solidified metal droplets that are left on the machined surfaces following the electrical discharge machining process. Following corrosion testing, a notable difference in corrosion resistance was observed between the samples. Sample 13, depicted in Fig. 6.5b, c demonstrated minimal corrosion damage, suggesting effective protection against corrosive elements. Its surface retained much of its original integrity, indicating a robust resistance to environmental factors. In contrast, Sample 8, shown in Fig. 6.5e, f exhibited significant surface degradation. This sample was marked by pronounced surface deterioration that included severe irregularities, extensive pitting, and the formation of microcracks. Such deterioration suggests a considerable weakness in corrosion resistance, highlighting the impact of the machining process on long-term performance under corrosive conditions [3–6].

An additional experiment was conducted on the Co–Cr alloy to investigate its corrosion resistance using the optimal processing parameters established through ANOVA analysis. The specific settings employed in this experiment included a

Table 6.4 Corrosion parameters calculated by the Tafel extrapolation method

Trial No.	E_{corr} (mV)	I_{corr} (A/cm^2)	Corrosion rate (mm/year)	Polarization resistance (Ω)
Untreated	– 136.26	181.26 n	0.002025	386.680 k
1	– 63.482	268.29 n	0.002961	367.400 k
2	– 85.998	3.6162 μ	0.039954	81.3850 k
3	– 275.04	2.7351 μ	0.030189	60.6150 k
4	– 99.783	1.9406 μ	0.021433	69.5880 k
5	– 34.493	52.6580 n	0.000581	1.54370 M
6	– 37.359	507.960 n	0.005607	99.9150 k
7	– 97.3	1.64960 μ	0.018208	84.0300 k
8	– 275.93	5.4435 μ	0.060112	33.5240 k
9	– 86.131	97.8660 n	0.001080	971.540 k
10	– 128.95	1.42700 μ	0.015751	109.160 k
11	– 127.52	2.20670 μ	0.024358	95.1140 k
12	– 134.76	1.74640 μ	0.019277	94.18880 k
13	– 120.27	35.1150 n	0.000388	2.67740 M
14	– 114.68	1.87006 μ	0.020649	89.4980 k
15	– 146.12	1.18180 μ	0.013052	98.9140 k
16	– 158.25	1.80660 μ	0.019941	94.9710 k
17	– 125.14	1.13600 μ	0.012539	132.390 k
18	– 84.957	390.001 n	0.004305	1.57560 M

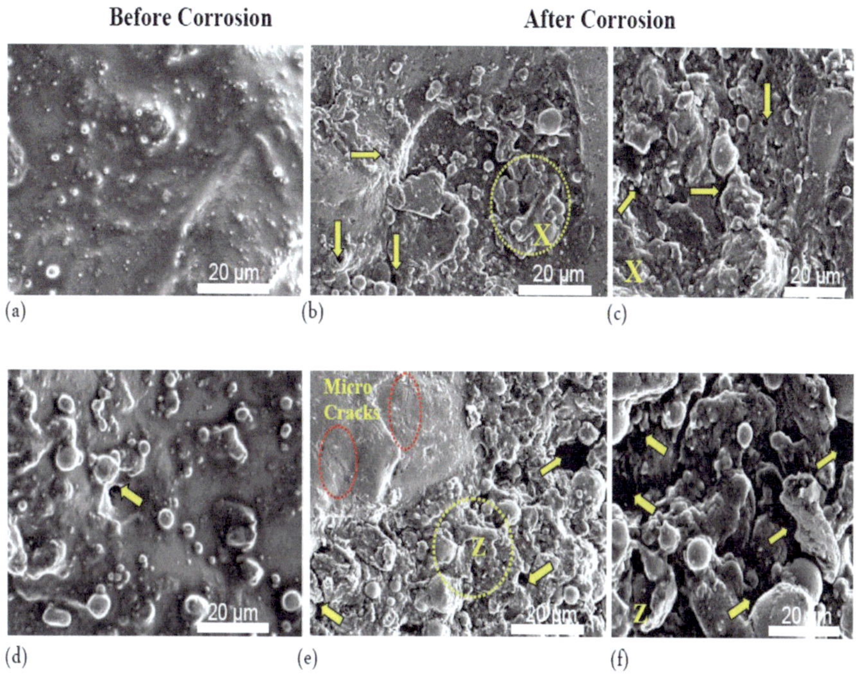

Fig. 6.5 SEM images from Sample 13 (**a–c**) and Sample 8 (**d–f**) treated surfaces before and after corrosion testing. Both surfaces demonstrate rough, porous grain with distinctive melting drops (mark (arrow): → corresponds to porous texture and melting drops; magnified at X and Z). After corrosion testing, Sample 13 shows low surface irregularities as compared to Sample 8. Reproduced with permission from Springer Nature [1]

current of 10 A, a pulse-on time of 200 µs, and a pulse-off time of 60 µs, utilizing a tungsten-copper (W–Cu) electrode submerged in deionized water to ensure a controlled environment. In Fig. 6.6, we present a detailed comparison of the corrosion rates observed in Sample 13 versus the sample machined using the optimal parameters. The results indicate that the optimally processed sample exhibits significantly enhanced corrosion resistance. Specifically, this sample demonstrated a corrosion rate of 0.00029 mm/year, which is notably lower than the corrosion rate recorded for Sample 13. This improvement underscores the effectiveness of the selected parameters in enhancing the material's durability and resistance to corrosive environments, further highlighting the importance of precise machining conditions in material performance.

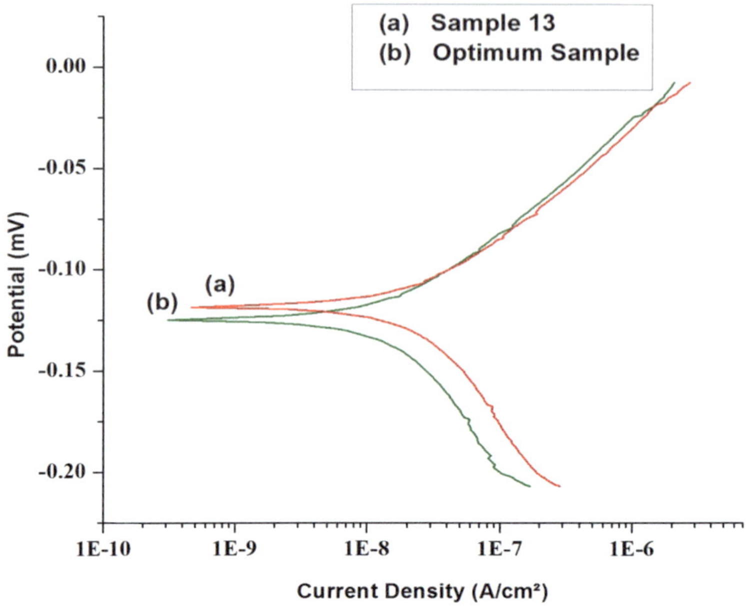

Fig. 6.6 Potentiodynamic polarization curves of **a** Sample 13; **b** optimum parameters machined sample

6.2.3 Hemocompatibility Analysis

Samples that showed exceptional corrosion resistance, specifically, Trials 13, 5, and 9, were thoroughly evaluated for their hemolysis behavior. This evaluation is important as hemolysis refers to the breakdown of red blood cells, which is crucial for assessing the biocompatibility of materials intended for medical use. In our tests, Triton X^{TM}-100 was employed as a positive control, and it resulted in complete hemolysis, showing a rate of 100%. Conversely, the negative control, consisting of phosphate-buffered saline (PBS) at pH 7.4, exhibited a minimal hemolysis rate of 4.89 ± 2.01%. This figure establishes a baseline for expected hemolytic activity. The untreated sample demonstrated a significantly higher hemolysis rate of 44.65 ± 3.03%, markedly differing from the negative control with a *p*-value of less than 0.001. This result indicates that the untreated sample has poor compatibility with blood, which is a critical consideration in the development of bioactive materials. In contrast, Sample 13, which was treated using an electrical discharge method, exhibited markedly improved hemocompatibility. Its hemolysis rate did not show a statistically significant difference from the negative control, indicated by a *p*-value greater than 0.05. This suggests that this treatment significantly enhances the sample's compatibility with blood, making it a promising candidate for medical applications. On the other hand, Samples 5 and 9 display moderate hemolysis rates of 20.17 ± 4.51% and 24.15 ± 3.31%, respectively. Both rates were significantly higher than the

Table 6.5 Absorbance (Abs) and % hemolysis (% hem) responses

Trial No.	$N = 1$		$N = 2$		$N = 3$		% hem Avg. ± S.D.
	Abs	% hem	Abs	% hem	Abs	% hem	
5	0.065	17.10	0.056	18.06	0.071	25.35	20.17 ± 4.51
9	0.079	20.78	0.085	27.41	0.068	24.28	24.15 ± 3.31
13	0.051	13.42	0.036	11.6	0.025	8.9	11.3 ± 2.27
Untreated	0.18	47.36	0.140	45.16	0.116	41.42	44.65 ± 3.03
PBS (−ve control)	0.007	2.1	0.018	5.8	0.017	6.78	4.89 ± 2.01
Triton (+ve control)	0.380	100	0.310	100	0.28	100	100

Reproduced with permission from Springer Nature [1]
N = No. of attempts

negative control, with p-values less than 0.05, indicating that while they show some improvement over the untreated sample, they still have a considerable hemolytic response that may limit their usability in clinical settings.

The absorbance (Abs) values, along with the corresponding percentages of hemolysis for each sample, are detailed in Table 6.5. To further validate the findings related to hemolysis, an examination of red blood cell morphology was conducted using a biological microscope, with the results presented in Fig. 6.7. Sample 13 exhibited remarkably minimal hemolysis, characterized by a significantly higher concentration of intact RBCs remaining undamaged. In contrast, the untreated sample showed pronounced clumping, accumulation, and deformation of the RBCs, indicative of severe hemolytic activity. Such alterations in the morphology of the RBCs underscore the detrimental effects of the untreated condition [7–9]. Moreover, Samples 5 and 9 displayed improvements in RBC morphology compared to the untreated specimen, suggesting a positive influence on cell integrity. In particular, Sample 9 manifested noticeable signs of protein agglomeration on the surfaces of the RBCs, which was evident in the microscopic images as a blurred background. This particular phenomenon of protein attachment could indicate interactions that may affect RBC functionality. Notably, this protein agglomeration was absent in Sample 13, further reinforcing its classification as a superior hemocompatible option based on the preserved morphology and minimal hemolysis observed.

6.2.4 XRD Analysis

The X-ray diffraction (XRD) patterns for the untreated surface and selected treated samples, specifically Samples 5, 8, and 13, are illustrated in Fig. 6.8. Each of these samples primarily contained elemental compounds such as chromium (Cr), nickel (Ni), molybdenum (Mo), and cobalt (Co), which are significant due to their well-known properties in enhancing material durability and corrosion resistance. Among the treated surfaces, Sample 5 exhibited remarkable corrosion resistance, which can

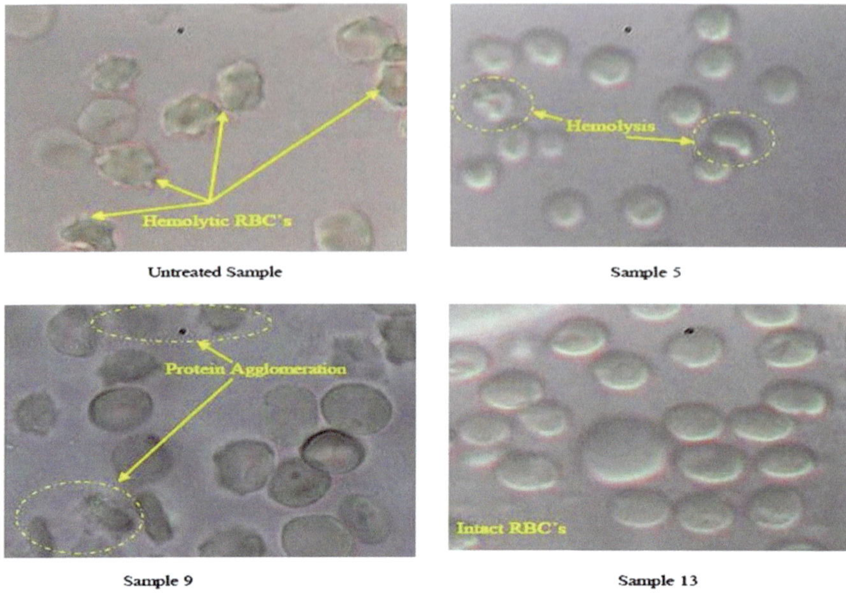

Fig. 6.7 RBC morphology of EDM-treated and untreated specimens. Reproduced with permission from Springer Nature [1]

be attributed to the formation of several specific surface phases. These include a tetragonal oxide (GeO_2), which is known for its stability and protection properties; an orthorhombic carbide (Cr_7C_3), which contributes to hardness and wear resistance; and a cubic boride ($B_6Co_{21}Mo_2$), recognized for its robust structural integrity [10, 11]. This combination of phases creates a protective layer that effectively mitigates corrosive attacks. In contrast, Sample 13 displayed a thin oxide layer composed of cubic beryllium oxide (Be_1O_1) and monoclinic phosphorus nitride ($N_1O_1P_1$). The presence of these phases, along with an increased oxygen content, is hypothesized to enhance its corrosion protection capabilities and improve the bioactivity of the implant material [2, 12]. Such bioactive characteristics are particularly important in biomedical applications, as they may improve the integration of implants with biological tissues. On the other hand, Sample 8 presented a significantly different profile, showcasing the presence of hexagonal vanadium and cubic yttrium-based phases. These phases are typically linked to elevated corrosion rates due to their inadequate protective properties [13–15]. The absence of a stable oxide layer on this sample is a crucial factor that further elucidates its poor corrosion resistance when compared to the more resilient samples. This differential behavior underscores the importance of phase composition and surface treatment in the performance of materials exposed to corrosive environments.

This investigation aimed to evaluate the electrochemical corrosion resistance and hemocompatibility of medical-grade cobalt-chromium (Co–Cr) alloys, which are widely used in biomedical applications due to their desirable mechanical properties

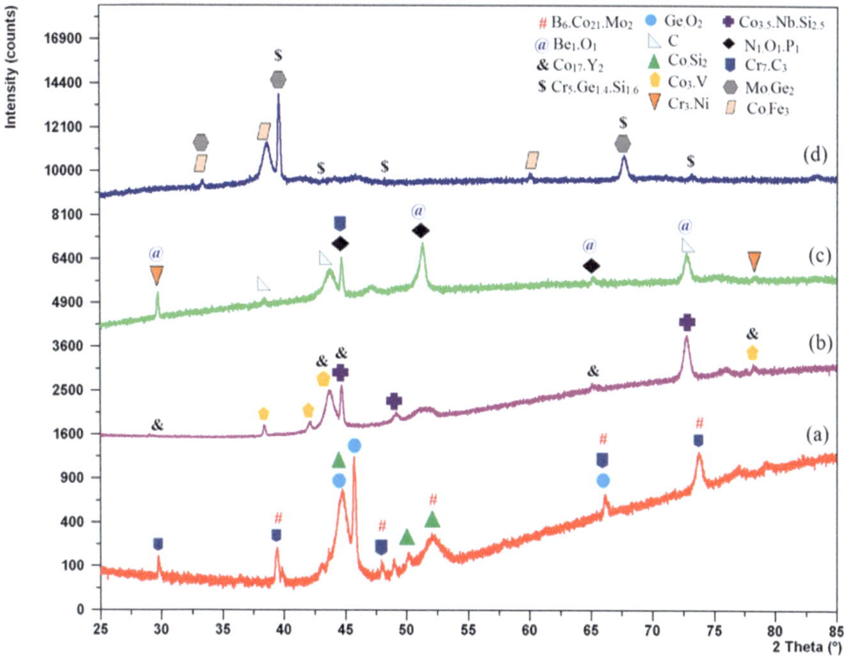

Fig. 6.8 XRD pattern of Co–Cr specimen **a** Trial 5, **b** Trial 8, **c** Trial 13, **d** untreated surface. Reproduced with permission from Springer Nature [1]

and biocompatibility. To assess the corrosion behavior of these alloys, we employed potentiodynamic polarization curves, which allowed us to accurately determine the corrosion potential and current density for each sample tested. Among all the samples examined, including both untreated and those processed using EDM, Sample 13 demonstrated the highest level of corrosion resistance. This sample recorded an impressive corrosion current density (I_{corr}) of 35.1150 nA/cm^2 and a remarkably low corrosion rate of just 0.0003 mm/year, highlighting its suitability for long-term applications in medical environments where longevity and reliability are critical. We compared our findings on corrosion resistance with those of previous studies to contextualize the performance of our Co–Cr alloy samples. For example, research conducted by Yang et al. [16] revealed that adding 2 mass% copper to Co–Cr alloys significantly improved their corrosion resistance, reporting an I_{corr} of 3.40 μA/cm^2. In another study, Tuna et al. [17] found that Co–Cr samples fabricated using advanced techniques like CAD/CAM milling and laser sintering exhibited superior corrosion resistance, measured at $I_{corr} = 16.88\ \mu$A/cm^2, compared to those produced through conventional casting methods, which tend to have higher porosity and defects that can compromise corrosion resistance. Furthermore, Qiu et al. [18] conducted experiments that showed a slight decrease in corrosion current density after subjecting Co–Cr alloys to a simulated porcelain firing process. This suggests that certain manufacturing processes may influence the electrochemical properties of Co–Cr alloys, reinforcing the need for careful selection of manufacturing techniques to optimize the performance of these crucial biomaterials in clinical applications. Overall, our study adds valuable insights into the factors affecting the corrosion resistance of Co–Cr alloys, offering guidance for their use in various medical applications.

6.3 Conclusions

The surface of cobalt-chromium (Co–Cr) alloy substrates was modified through a process known as EDT, which is electrical discharge treatment, to evaluate their corrosion characteristics and hemocompatibility using detailed electrochemical analysis. The findings demonstrated significant enhancement in both corrosion resistance and blood compatibility for the EDM-treated samples compared to their untreated counterparts. In particular, the study highlighted that EDM-treated Sample 13 provided superior corrosion protection, outperforming the other tested substrates. The electrochemical analysis revealed that Sample 13 not only resisted corrosion more effectively but also exhibited intriguing improvements in its interaction with biological components. When assessing hemocompatibility, the EDM-treated surface of Sample 13 showed minimal signs of hemolysis and a significantly greater quantity of intact red blood cells (RBCs) in comparison to the untreated sample. In the untreated substrate, RBCs appeared clumped, aggregated, and displayed noticeable morphological distortions, indicating poor compatibility with blood. Conversely, Samples 5 and 9 exhibited improved RBC structures, indicative of enhanced surface compatibility, although they did not match the performance of Sample 13. Additionally, when RBCs were exposed to the surface of Sample 9, microscopic analysis revealed an interesting phenomenon: protein agglomeration on the cell surfaces, which manifested as a blurred background in imaging. This occurrence suggested a potentially adverse interaction between the proteins in the blood and the surface characteristics of Sample 9. Notably, such protein agglomeration was absent in Sample 13, further corroborating its superior hemocompatibility and suggesting that it promotes a more favorable environment for blood components. Furthermore, statistical analysis using ANOVA identified the optimal parameters for the EDM process, which included a current of 10 A, a pulse-on time of 200 μs, a pulse-off time of 60 μs, and conducting the machining in deionized water using a tungsten-copper (W–Cu) electrode. These carefully controlled conditions yielded the most favorable surface characteristics, ultimately enhancing both the corrosion resistance and hemocompatibility of the Co–Cr alloy substrates. Thus, the study underscores the potential of EDM as a powerful technique for improving the performance of biomedical materials in applications where corrosion resistance and biocompatibility are critical.

References

1. Mahajan A, Sidhu SS (2019) In vitro corrosion and hemocompatibility evaluation of electrical discharge treated cobalt–chromium implant. J Mater Res 34(8):1363–1370
2. Chen Q, McEwen GD, Zaveri N, Karpagavalli R, Zhou A (2012) Corrosion resistance of Ti–6Al–4V with nanostructured TiO_2 coatings. Emerg Nanotechnol Dentist 165–179
3. Mahajan A, Devgan S, Sidhu SS (2021) Surface alteration of biomedical alloys by electrical discharge treatment for enhancing the electrochemical corrosion, tribological and biological performances. Surf Coat Technol 405:126583
4. Singh G, Sidhu SS, Bains PS, Singh M, Bhui AS (2020) On surface modification of Ti alloy by electro discharge coating using hydroxyapatite powder mixed dielectric with graphite tool. J Bio- Tribo-Corros 6(3):91
5. Mahajan A, Devgan S (2025) Recent advances in surface engineering of additive manufactured materials for enhancing corrosion resistance. Prog Addit Manuf 10(2):1103–1118
6. Okokpujie IP, Tartibu LK, Musa-Basheer HO, Adeoye AOM (2024) Effect of coatings on mechanical, corrosion and tribological properties of industrial materials: a comprehensive review. J Bio- Tribo-Corros 10(1):2
7. Devgan S, Mahajan A, Singh G, Singh G, Sidhu SS (2021) Surface integrity of powder mixed electrical discharge treated substrate at high discharge energies. In: Sustainable machining strategies for better performance: select proceedings of SMSBP 2020. Springer Singapore, Singapore, pp 207–217
8. McNamee AP, Simmonds MJ (2023) Red blood cell sublethal damage: hemocompatibility is not the absence of hemolysis. Transfus Med Rev 37(2):150723
9. Rakshak R, Bhatt S, Sharma S, Agharkar R, Bodakhe S, Srivastava R (2024) Characterizing morphological alterations in blood related disorders through atomic force microscopy. Nanotheranostics 8(3):330
10. Yu LG, Khor KA, Sundararajan G (2006) Boride layer growth kinetics during boriding of molybdenum by the spark plasma sintering (SPS) technology. Surf Coat Technol 201(6):2849–2853
11. Natesan K, Johnson RN (1987) Corrosion resistance of chromium carbide coatings in oxygen-sulfur environments. Surf Coat Technol 33:341–351
12. Im BM, Akiyama E, Habazaki H, Kawashima A, Asami K, Hashimoto K (1995) The effect of phosphorus addition on the corrosion behavior of amorphous Fe-8Cr-P alloys in 9M H_2SO_4. Corros Sci 37(5):709–722
13. Lai GY (2007) High-temperature corrosion and materials applications, 1st edn. ASM International, Ohio, USA, p 21
14. Mahajan A, Singh G, Devgan S, Sidhu SS (2021) EDM performance characteristics and electrochemical corrosion analysis of Co–Cr alloy and duplex stainless steel: a comparative study. Proc Inst Mech Eng Part E J Proc Mech Eng 235(4):812–823
15. Singh G, Singh M, Sidhu SS, Ablyaz TR (2022) Improving surface characteristics and corrosion resistance of medical grade 316L by titanium powder mixed electro-discharge treatment. Surf Topogr Metrol Prop 10(2):025002
16. Yang B, Shi C, Li Y, Lei Q, Nie Y (2018) Effect of Cu on the corrosion resistance and electrochemical response of a Ni–Co–Cr–Mo alloy in acidic chloride solution. J Mater Res 33(22):3801–3808
17. Tuna SH, Pekmez NO, Kurkçuoglu I (2015) Corrosion resistance assessment of Co–Cr alloy frameworks fabricated by CAD/CAM milling, laser sintering, and casting methods. J Prosthet Dent 114(5):725–734
18. Qiu J, Yu WQ, Zhang FQ, Smales RJ, Zhang YL, Lu CH (2011) Corrosion behaviour and surface analysis of a Co–Cr and two Ni–Cr dental alloys before and after simulated porcelain firing. Eur J Oral Sci 119(1):93–101

Chapter 7
Tribological Performance Analysis of Co–Cr Alloy (Stage III)

This chapter provides an in-depth evaluation of the effectiveness of EDM in enhancing the tribological performance and cytocompatibility of medical-grade cobalt-chromium (Co–Cr) alloy. EDM is a crucial process in the manufacturing of metallic implants, as it can significantly influence both the mechanical properties and biological compatibility of the materials used. For this study, the most effective EDM process parameters identified in earlier stages (Stages I and II) were selected for further analysis. These parameters are vital for optimizing the performance of metallic implants in biomedical applications. The Co–Cr specimens used in this research were subjected to treatment using a tungsten-copper (W–Cu) electrode within a deionized water tank, serving as the dielectric medium. Different spark energy levels were applied during the EDM process, allowing for a comprehensive investigation of their effects on the material's properties. To evaluate the cytocompatibility of the modified substrates, the MTT assay was conducted. This assay is a well-established method that measures cell viability by assessing the metabolic activity of cells after exposure to the substrates. By analyzing the results of the MTT assay, we can determine how well the material supports cell growth and proliferation, which is crucial for successful implantation. In addition to cytocompatibility, the wear rate and coefficient of friction of the substrates were assessed using a pin-on-disk tribometer. This method provides valuable insights into the tribological performance of the Co–Cr alloy, specifically its resistance to wear and friction under simulated physiological conditions. The experimental setup and operational parameters of the EDM machine are illustrated in Fig. 7.1, providing a visual reference for the arrangement used throughout the study. This comprehensive approach allows for a thorough understanding of how EDM treatments can optimize Co–Cr alloys for medical applications, ensuring both durability and biocompatibility in implantable devices.

© The Author(s), under exclusive license to Springer Nature Singapore Pte Ltd. 2026
A. Mahajan et al., *Surface Modification of Co–Cr Alloy for Orthopaedic Applications*, Biomedical Materials for Multi-functional Applications,
https://doi.org/10.1007/978-981-95-4029-7_7

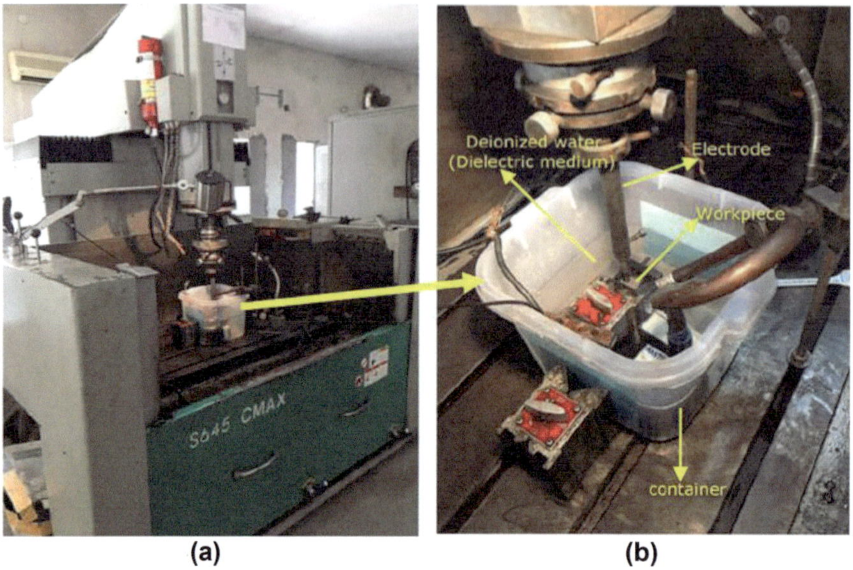

Fig. 7.1 **a** EDM machine and **b** experimental setup of EDM. Reproduced with permission from Springer Nature [1]

7.1 Selection of Parameters for Experimentation of Stage III

The machining parameters for Stage III were meticulously developed based on the insights and results obtained from the earlier Phase I and Phase II experiments, as illustrated in Fig. 7.2. During Stage II, specific electrical discharge machining settings were identified that showed optimal performance in terms of corrosion resistance and hemocompatibility, key factors for ensuring the material's suitability in medical applications. For Stage III, the second sample was meticulously selected from the L18 orthogonal array utilized in Stage II. This selection was based on its spark energy level, which precisely aligned with the biocompatible range determined during Phase I. This ensures that the machining process contributes positively to the material's properties without compromising safety or effectiveness for biomedical purposes. Additionally, for the third set of parameters, we opted for the lowest discharge current available. This was paired with the same pulse-on time that had been effectively used in both the first and second samples. This choice was made to explore how a lower discharge current could further enhance the machined surface quality. The configuration implemented for testing was conducted in deionized water, which served as the dielectric medium. This choice was fundamental, as it was also derived from the experimental design established in Stage II, ensuring continuity and comparability in results across the different stages of the study.

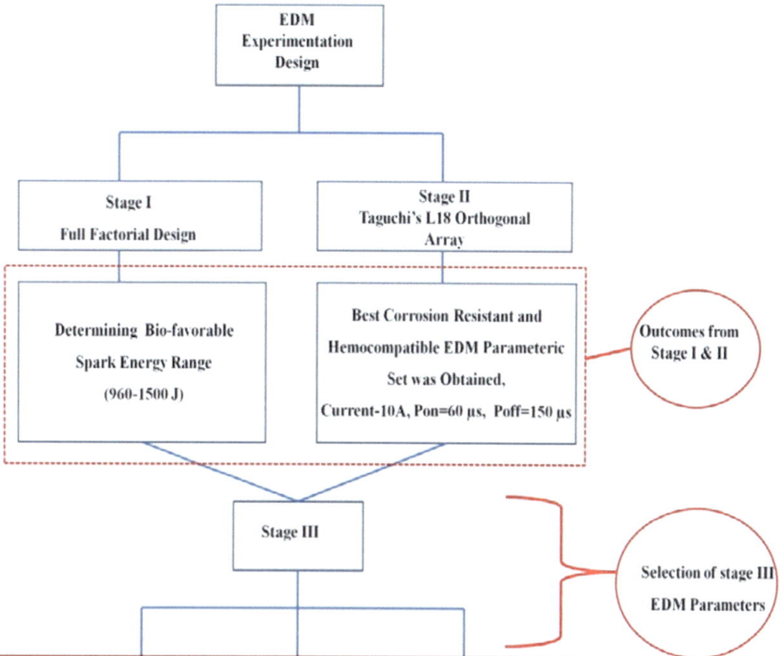

Input Factors	Trial 1	Trial 2	Trial 3
Current (A)	5	10	16
Pulse on Time (μs)	60	60	60
Pulse off Time(μs)	200	150	200
Voltage(V)	140		
Electrode	Tungsten Copper (W-Cu)		
Dielectric Medium	Deionized Water		

Fig. 7.2 Selection of Stage III EDM process parameters

7.1.1 Pin-On-Disk Wear Study

Wear testing of the Co–Cr alloy specimens was conducted using an advanced pin-on-disk tribometer, manufactured by DUCOM Instruments in Bangalore, India, as illustrated in Fig. 7.3. This method is widely recognized for its ability to simulate friction and wear in materials under controlled conditions. Comprehensive specifications of the tribometer setup, including the operational parameters and calibration details, can be found in Table 7.1. The tribometer featured a disk made of EN31 steel, a highly durable material known for its wear resistance, measuring 120 mm in diameter and 10 mm in thickness. The Co–Cr alloy samples were precisely shaped into pin configurations, achieved through a soldering process utilizing the same alloy material, resulting in pins that were 45 mm long and 10 mm in diameter. Ringer's solution was employed as the lubricating medium during the tests; this physiological saline solution is commonly used in tribological studies due to its effective lubrication properties and compatibility with biological materials. To ensure accurate results, the primary wear track diameter on the disk was maintained at 80 mm throughout the testing process. A consistent normal load of 70 N was applied to each pin, simulating realistic loading conditions, and the disk was rotated at a steady speed of 100 rpm to replicate typical wear scenarios. Each wear test was carried out for a duration of 3600 s, allowing sufficient time to observe the material's behavior under friction. Before and after each testing session, both the wear tracks on the disk and the pin specimens were meticulously cleaned with acetone to remove any debris or contaminants that could affect the results. To validate the findings and ensure repeatability, all tests were conducted three times ($n = 3$) under controlled room temperature conditions. This rigorous methodology highlights the reliability of the wear testing process and the precision involved in studying the performance of Co–Cr alloy materials in tribological applications.

The operational parameters, including speed, load, and temperature, were monitored and analyzed alongside the wear and friction measurements between the pin and disk. This was achieved using an advanced computer system integrated with TR-20LE software, which facilitated real-time data collection and analysis. To assess

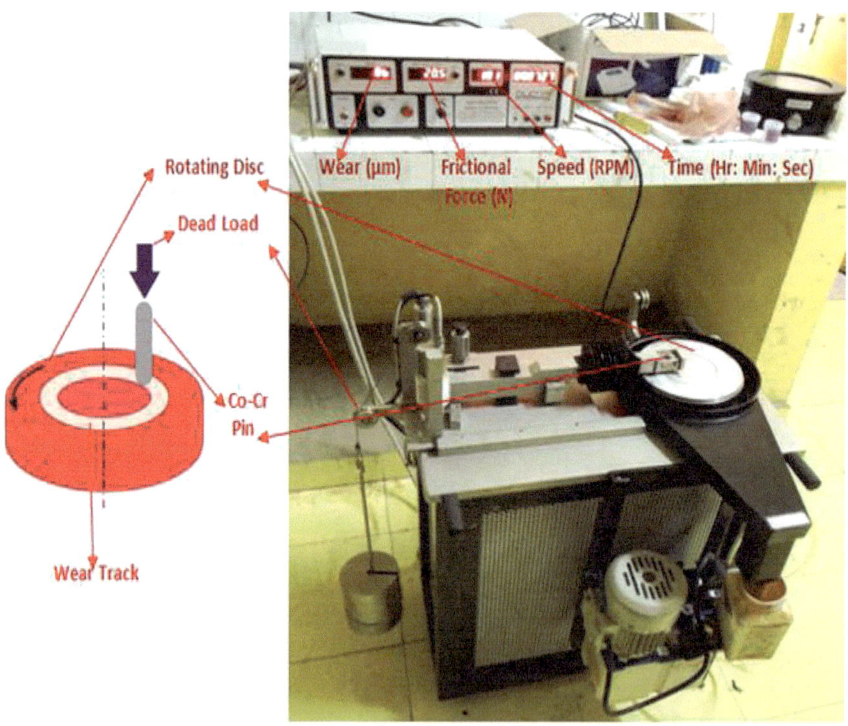

Fig. 7.3 Pictorial and schematic view of the pin-on-disk apparatus. Reproduced with permission from Springer Nature [1]

Table 7.1 Specification of pin-on-disk tribometer (DUCOM)

Parameters	Values
Pin size	3, 5, 10, and 12 mm (in diameter)
Disk diameter	100–200 mm
Disk rotation speed	0–2950 rpm
Wear track diameter mean	50–100 mm
Load	5–200 N
Sliding speed range	0–10 m/s
Frictional force	0–200 N
Wear measurement	0–2000 μm (1 μm LC)
Temperature	Ambient to 300 °C
Power	230 V, 50 Hz S phase

the wear behavior of the material, the wear rate (W.R.) was calculated, expressed in mm^3/Nm. This was determined using the mass loss method, a reliable technique that involves measuring the decrease in mass of the tested specimens after exposure to the operational conditions. The following equation (Eq. 7.1) was employed for this calculation, providing a quantitative assessment of wear performance under varying operational scenarios:

$$\text{W.R.} = \frac{\Delta m}{L * \rho * W} \tag{7.1}$$

where

- Δm represents the mass loss in grams,
- L is the total sliding distance in meters,
- ρ denotes the density of pin material (for Co–Cr material: $\rho = 8.3$ g/mm^3) and
- W is the applied load in Newtons.

The mass loss of the pins was measured using a high-precision electronic balance produced by Saffron Electronic Scale, located in Gujarat, India. This advanced instrument is designed to provide exceptional accuracy, with a measurement precision of ± 0.1 mg. The careful calibration of the balance ensured reliable data collection, which is crucial for understanding the structural integrity and performance characteristics of the pins during the experiment.

7.1.2 *In-Vitro Cytocompatibility Test*

To evaluate the cellular response to EDMed surfaces, comprehensive in-vitro cytotoxicity assessments were conducted as per the established protocol outlined in Stage I of our study. During this phase, we specifically assessed the cytotoxic effects of the fabricated specimens using the MTT assay, which is a colorimetric assay that measures cell viability based on the reduction of 3-(4,5-Dimethylthiazol-2-yl)-2,5-Diphenyltetrazolium Bromide (MTT) to formazan crystals by metabolically active cells. The MG-63 human osteosarcoma cell line, obtained from the National Centre for Cell Science (NCCS) in Pune, India, was utilized for this experiment. This cell line serves as a valuable model for studying bone cancer and provides insights into cellular response mechanisms. Through this evaluation, we aimed to gain a deeper understanding of how the EDMed surfaces interact with human osteosarcoma cells, specifically regarding their cytotoxic potential.

To gain a deeper understanding of the surface wear characteristics of the electrically discharged machined (EDMed) samples, we employed Field Emission Scanning Electron Microscopy (FESEM) using a Hitachi SU-8010 instrument, which is based in Tokyo, Japan. This advanced microscopy technique allows for high-resolution imaging of the sample surfaces, enabling us to identify and analyze various wear features in detail. In addition to the surface analysis, we assessed cellular toxicity qualitatively through microscopic observation of cells exposed to these samples. This assessment is critical for evaluating the biocompatibility of the materials under investigation. Furthermore, we conducted an MTT assay, a colorimetric assay for assessing cell metabolic activity, to determine cell viability. The layout of the 24-well plate, which illustrates the arrangement of the samples and control conditions used during the assay, is detailed in Fig. 7.4. This figure serves as a visual reference to the experimental setup and aids in understanding the context of the results derived from the study.

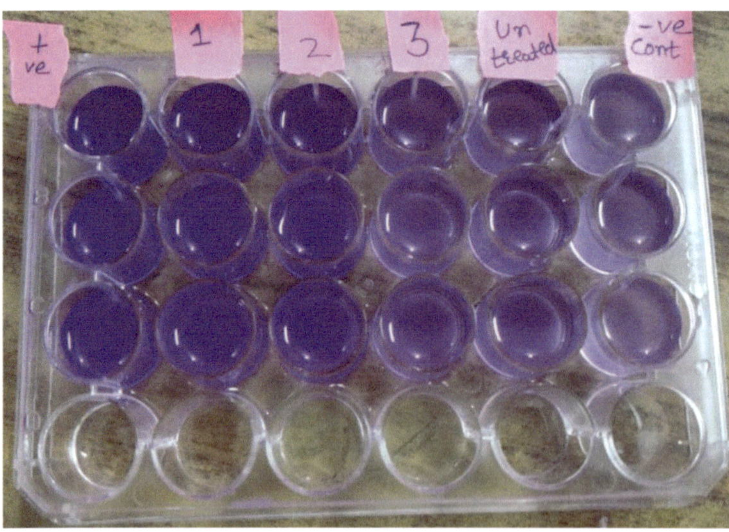

Fig. 7.4 Well plate after MTT assay—dark purple color represented a large number of cells. Reproduced with permission from Springer Nature [1]

7.2 Results and Discussion

This experimental study aimed to thoroughly investigate the effectiveness of EDM in enhancing both the cytocompatibility and tribological behavior of medical-grade Cobalt-Chromium (Co–Cr) alloy, which is widely used in biomedical applications. The focus of the research was to determine how various machining parameters influence the material properties relevant to medical implants. As outlined in the previous sections, the machining parameters for Stage III were carefully developed based on the findings from Stages I and II. These earlier stages provided critical insights into how adjustments in EDM settings could impact the alloy's performance in terms of biocompatibility and wear resistance. A summary of the selected parameters for Stage III, along with their expected effects, can be found in Table 7.2. This structured approach allows for a systematic evaluation of the EDM process and its implications for the future development of advanced materials in the medical field.

7.2.1 Cytocompatibility Analysis

The cytotoxic response of both untreated and EDMed specimens was rigorously assessed by measuring the percentage viability of MG63 osteosarcoma cells. The analysis revealed that the negative control group, which consisted of cells cultured on a standard glass coverslip, exhibited a significantly higher cell viability compared to the cobalt-chromium (Co–Cr) alloy samples, with a statistical significance level of $p < 0.001$. In particular, Samples 3 (EDM-treated) and the untreated specimen showed no statistically significant differences in cell viability when compared to the positive control (CPT), indicated by a p-value greater than 0.05. This suggests that the cytotoxic effects on these samples were comparable to the positive control condition. Conversely, Samples 1 and 2 demonstrated significantly enhanced cell viability, with percentages ranging from 80 to 88%, accompanied by a statistical significance level of $p < 0.05$. Notably, Sample 2 exhibited an impressive approximately 1.9-fold increase in MG63 cell viability when compared to the unmachined sample, highlighting its superior biocompatibility. Comprehensive data regarding the percentage cell viability

Table 7.2 Input parameters and their values for Stage III

Input factors	Sample 1	Sample 2	Sample 3
Current (A)	5	10	16
Pulse on time (μs)	60	60	60
Pulse pause time (μs)	200	150	200
Voltage (V)	140		
Electrode	Tungsten copper (W–Cu)		
Dielectric medium	Deionized water		

Reproduced with permission from Springer Nature [1]

and absorbance (Abs) values for all tested and untreated specimens are meticulously summarized in Table 7.3. Additionally, a visual representation depicting the behavior of cell toxicity in response to interaction with the different samples is illustrated in Fig. 7.5, offering valuable insights into the effects of the materials on cellular health.

Comparable trends were observed in the morphological analysis of MG63 cells through detailed microscopic imaging, as illustrated in Fig. 7.6. Among the samples, the negative control exhibited the highest concentration of viable cells, indicating a robust cell population with healthy characteristics. Samples 1 and 2, which had previously demonstrated elevated cell viability percentages, also showed a dense aggregation of adherent, healthy cells when examined under the microscope. This suggests not only high viability but also effective attachment, which is crucial for successful integration in biomedical applications. In stark contrast, both the untreated

Table 7.3 Absorbance (Abs) and % cell viability (% Via) of testing samples

Specimen name	$N = 1$		$N = 2$		$N = 3$		% Via Average ± S.D.
	Abs	% Via	Abs	% Via	Abs	% Via	
Sample 1	0.657	81.81	0.642	80.55	0.632	82.50	81.62 ± 0.98
Sample 2	0.701	87.29	0.686	86.07	0.676	88.25	87.20 ± 1.09
Sample 3	0.378	47.07	0.365	45.79	0.389	50.78	47.88 ± 2.59
Untreated	0.337	41.96	0.344	43.16	0.371	48.43	44.52 ± 3.44
CPT (+ve control)	0.292	36.36	0.287	36.01	0.291	37.98	36.78 ± 1.05
DMEM (−ve control)	0.803	100	0.797	100	0.766	100	100

Reproduced with permission from Springer Nature [1]
N = No. of attempts

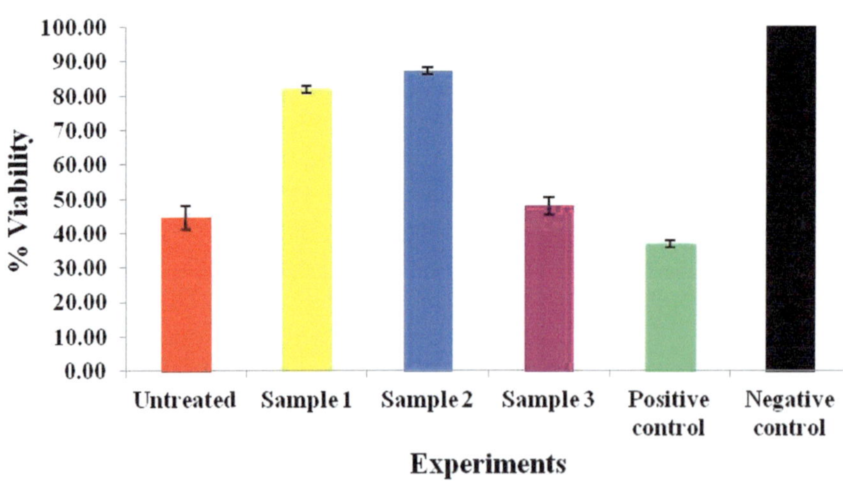

Fig. 7.5 Percentage cell viability upon samples. All values expressed as Average ± S.D., at n = 3. Reproduced with permission from Springer Nature [1]

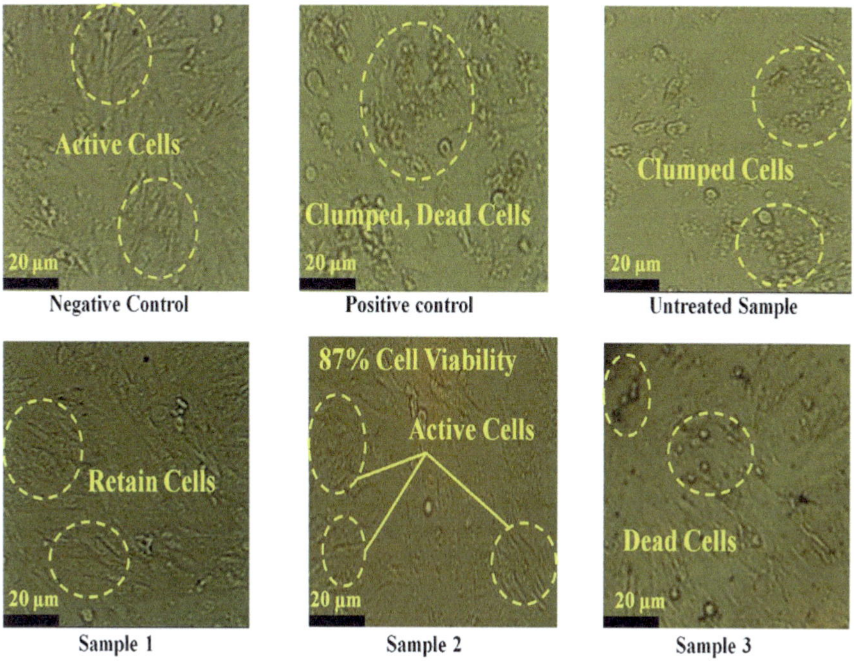

Fig. 7.6 Microscope images represent cytotoxicity response upon the samples. Reproduced with permission from Springer Nature [1]

control sample and Sample 3 displayed a significant presence of dead or deteriorated cells. The morphology of these two samples closely resembled that of the positive control group, which is typically indicative of detriment to cell health and functionality [2–4]. These findings are consistent with the quantitative cell viability data, reinforcing the conclusion that EDM-treated samples, especially Samples 1 and 2, exhibit significantly improved biocompatibility compared to the unmachined surface. The favorable characteristics observed in Samples 1 and 2 provide compelling evidence for the potential application of EDM-treated implants in biomedical fields, as they show promise in promoting cell survival and adhesion. Conversely, the underperformance of Sample 3 underscores the need for further investigation into optimization options for EDM treatment processes to enhance cell viability outcomes [5, 6].

7.2.2 Tribological Examination of EDMed Surfaces

Tables 7.4 and 7.5 provide a comprehensive overview of the measured values for both the coefficient of friction and the wear rates of each specimen tested in the study. Among the various samples analyzed, Sample 3 stood out with the highest wear rate, recorded at approximately $(6.6 \pm 0.34) \times 10^{-7}$ mm^3/Nm. This increased wear rate suggests a significant loss of material under the testing conditions, indicating that Sample 3 may be less durable in applications where wear resistance is critical. In contrast, Sample 2 demonstrated remarkable wear resistance, achieving the lowest wear rate at approximately $(1.24 \pm 0.14) \times 10^{-7}$ mm^3/Nm. This result positions Sample 2 as the most wear-resistant option among the specimens tested in the pin-on-disk apparatus, highlighting its potential suitability for demanding tribological applications. Additionally, the wear rates of the untreated specimen and Sample 1 were found to be nearly identical, suggesting that both exhibit comparable tribological performance. This similarity indicates that the modifications applied to Sample 1 did not significantly enhance its wear resistance relative to the untreated specimen. Overall, these findings provide valuable insights into the performance characteristics of each sample, emphasizing the importance of material selection in applications subject to wear and friction.

Figure 7.7a provides a detailed illustration of the relationship between wear, measured in micrometers (μm), and the corresponding time intervals, recorded in seconds, for the selected specimens. This data highlights the wear characteristics of different materials under controlled testing conditions. In Fig. 7.7b, a comprehensive comparative analysis of wear rates is presented for all tested samples, allowing for a clearer understanding of the performance of each material. Further insights into the performance of each pin specimen over time can be found in Fig. 7.7c, which depicts the variation in the coefficient of friction. Among the specimens tested, Sample 3 achieved the highest average coefficient of friction ($\mu \approx 0.37$), indicating greater resistance during sliding contact. In contrast, Sample 1 demonstrated the lowest

Table 7.4 Evaluated the coefficient of friction of the samples

Specimen name	$N = 1$	$N = 2$	$N = 3$	Average ± S.D.
	Coefficient of friction			
Untreated	0.317	0.309	0.312	0.313 ± 0.003
Sample 1	0.262	0.271	0.252	0.261 ± 0.009
Sample 2	0.294	0.3	0.289	0.291 ± 0.01
Sample 3	0.374	0.39	0.35	0.371 ± 0.02

Reproduced with permission from Springer Nature [1]

Table 7.5 Calculated wear rate of the specimens

Specimen name	$N = 1$	$N = 2$	$N = 3$	Average ± S.D.
	Wear rate (mm^3/Nm)			
Untreated	4.82×10^{-7}	4.96×10^{-7}	4.99×10^{-7}	$(4.93 \pm 0.09) \times 10^{-7}$
Sample 1	4.54×10^{-7}	4.74×10^{-7}	4.84×10^{-7}	$(4.71 \pm 0.15) \times 10^{-7}$
Sample 2	1.23×10^{-7}	1.25×10^{-7}	1.26×10^{-7}	$(1.24 \pm 0.14) \times 10^{-7}$
Sample 3	6.61×10^{-7}	6.96×10^{-7}	6.28×10^{-7}	$(6.67 \pm 0.34) \times 10^{-7}$

Reproduced with permission from Springer Nature [1]

average friction coefficient ($\mu \approx 0.26$), suggesting smoother interaction and potentially better lubricative properties. Notably, both the untreated sample and Sample 2 began the tests with nearly identical initial friction values, which signifies comparable surface characteristics before significant wear occurred. As the testing progressed, a gradual increase in friction was observed for both the untreated sample and Sample 2. The friction for the untreated sample rose from an initial value of 0.28–0.31, while Sample 2 experienced a slight increase from 0.27 to 0.29. This trend indicates a modest change in the surface interaction behavior over time, possibly linked to the wear processes affecting the surfaces. Such findings emphasize the importance of monitoring frictional behavior in relation to material wear, providing valuable insights for optimizing material selection in applications where wear resistance is critical.

The surface morphology of both untreated and EDT-treated samples prior to wear testing is depicted in Fig. 7.8a–d. The untreated specimen, provided by the supplier, displayed inherent micropores on its surface, as illustrated in Fig. 7.8a. These micropores are indicative of the material's initial state and suggest potential vulnerabilities for wear. In contrast, Sample 1, which was machined using a discharge current of 5 A

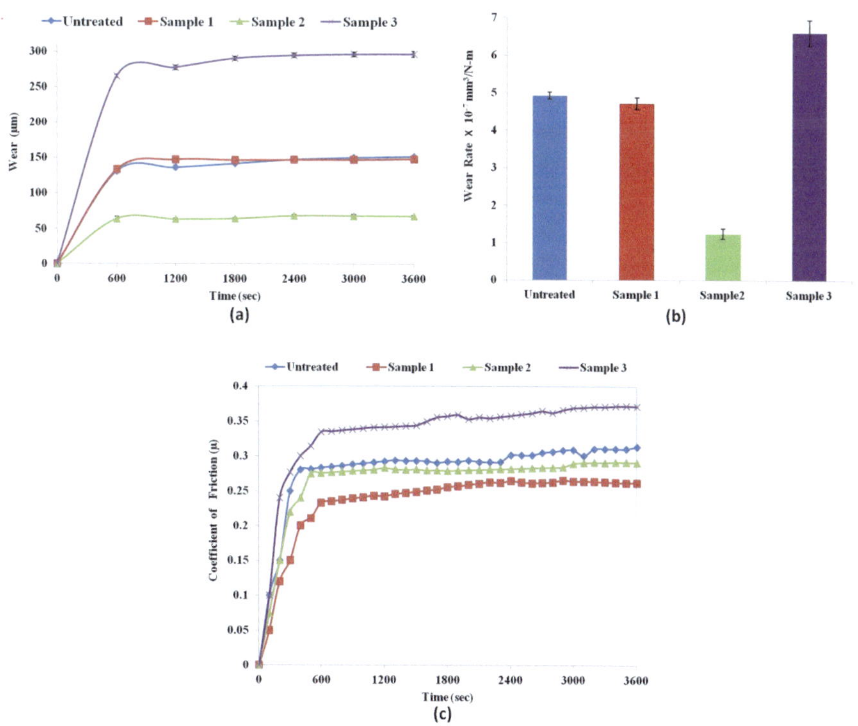

Fig. 7.7 **a** Variation of wear (µm) with time of pin samples; **b** wear rate comparison of samples; **c** variation of the coefficient of friction (μ) with time of pin samples. Reproduced with permission from Springer Nature [1]

and a pulse duration of 60 μs, exhibited significant surface features such as craters and small pores, as shown in Fig. 7.8b. The presence of these features suggests that the machining process enhanced the surface complexity, possibly affecting its tribological behavior. Sample 2, processed under similar pulse duration but with a higher current of 10 A, demonstrated a more refined surface morphology that included micropores, shallow valleys, and minor peaks, as indicated in Fig. 7.8c. This superior surface texture can be attributed to the efficient coordination between spark energy and the flushing mechanism, which effectively removes machining debris during the machining process. The removal of debris is crucial in achieving a smoother surface finish, which is essential for enhancing wear resistance.

The cross-sectional FESEM image of Sample 2, displayed in Fig. 7.8(i), revealed a distinct recast layer. This layer formed as a result of the re-solidification of molten material ejected from both the workpiece and the electrode during the continual sparking inherent in EDM. The formation of this recast layer is significant, as it has been shown to improve the microhardness and overall wear resistance of the material by creating a hardened surface that can better withstand abrasive conditions. When the discharge current was raised to 16 A, the resultant higher spark energy resulted in a more irregular surface structure characterized by deeper craters, pronounced ridges, and partially resolidified metallic droplets, as depicted in Fig. 7.8d. This alteration in surface morphology due to increased energy input suggests a trade-off between surface roughness and potential wear characteristics. Post-wear analysis using FESEM, presented in Fig. 7.8e–h, illustrated that the untreated surface experienced significant damage during wear testing. The damage included delamination, which involves the separation of layers, flake formation, and minor surface scratches, as evidenced in Fig. 7.8e. These findings highlight the vulnerabilities of untreated surfaces under wear conditions and emphasize the need for processing techniques that enhance surface integrity and durability.

Dark patches were observed on the surfaces of both modified Sample 1 and Sample 2, which serve as clear indicators of tribochemical reactions resulting from material wear in an oxygen-rich environment. These reactions often occur when surfaces experience friction, leading to the formation of oxide layers. In the case of Sample 1, the surface exhibited significant damage characterized by prominent scratches, deep grooves, and clear signs of delamination. These features suggest a higher level of stress and wear experienced by Sample 1, as illustrated in Fig. 7.8f. The extent of the damage implies that this sample is less capable of withstanding wear, potentially affecting its performance in practical applications. On the other hand, Sample 2 demonstrated a remarkably different condition. It showed minimal surface deterioration, featuring fewer scratches and almost no signs of delamination. Instead, it displayed a uniform distribution of moderate tribochemical oxide layers across its surface, as shown in Fig. 7.8g. These protective oxide layers likely contributed to the enhanced wear resistance observed in Sample 2. This aligns with previous findings reported by Ikeuchi et al. [7] and Hesketh et al. [8], which highlight the importance of surface characteristics in improving the longevity and durability of materials. In contrast, Sample 3 revealed extensive surface damage characterized by large scratches, significant flaking, and an absence of any tribochemical oxide layers.

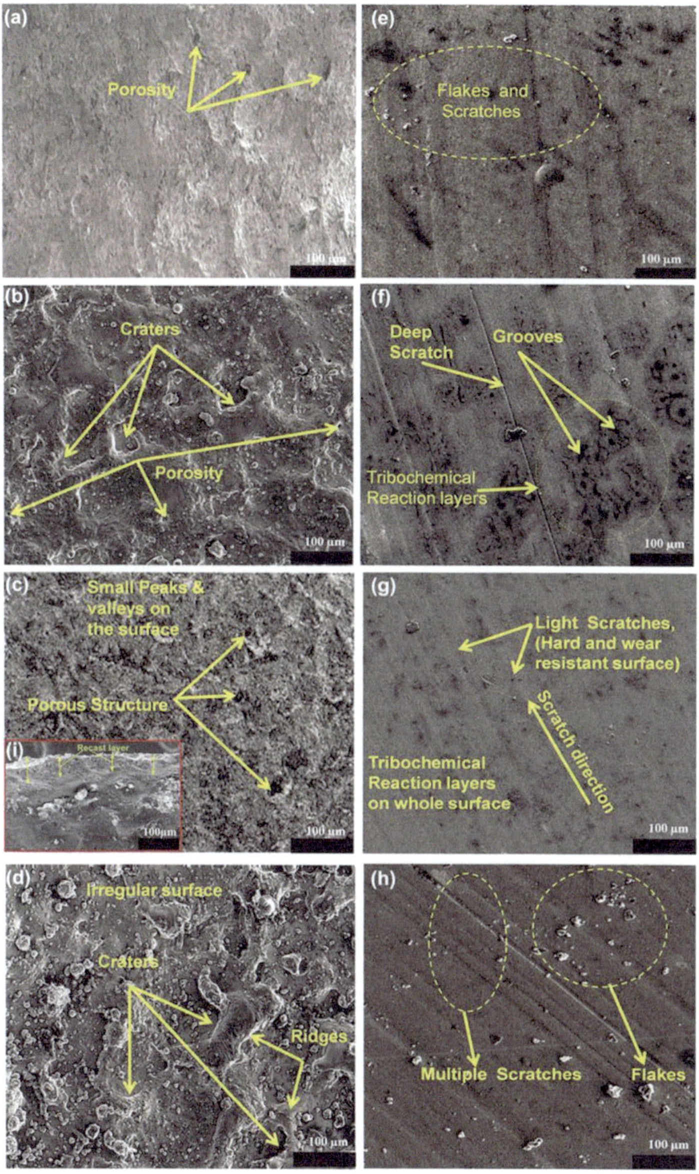

Fig. 7.8 FESEM images from untreated and treated substrates before (**a**–**d**) and after (**e**–**h**) wear testing. Before wear testing, **a** untreated substrate shows porous structure; **b**, **d** Sample 1 and Sample 3 surfaces demonstrate rough, porous grain with craters; **c** Sample 2 surface shows peaks, valleys, micropores along with suitable recast layer on its cross section (i). After wear testing, **e** untreated substrate demonstrate flakes, delaminations and small surface scratches; **f** worn surface of Sample 1 witnesses tribochemical layers, deep scratches, grooves, and delaminations; **g** Sample 2 affirms lesser scratches, no delaminations and tribochemical oxide layers on the whole surface; **h** Sample 3 exhibits multiple scratches and flakes. Reproduced with permission from Springer Nature [1]

This absence indicates a lack of protective mechanisms against wear, suggesting that Sample 3 is particularly susceptible to further degradation, as illustrated in Fig. 7.8h. The severe wear patterns observed in Sample 3 point to a need for improved material design or surface treatments to enhance its resistance to wear in environments similar to those tested.

To further validate the superior wear resistance exhibited by Sample 2, a comprehensive microhardness evaluation was performed. The findings revealed that Sample 2 achieved an impressive microhardness value of 773 HV0.2. This represents a substantial increase, approximately 1.75 times greater than the hardness of the untreated sample, which measured 442 HV0.2. The significant enhancement in microhardness not only underscores the effectiveness of the treatment applied to Sample 2 but also indicates a direct correlation with its improved wear performance. This improvement suggests that the structural integrity of Sample 2 is markedly better, making it more capable of withstanding wear under operational conditions.

7.2.3 EDX and XRD Analysis

The EDX analysis of both the untreated Sample 2 and its EDM-treated counterpart revealed promising outcomes regarding biocompatibility and wear performance, as illustrated in Fig. 7.9a, b. In both samples, the EDX analysis identified the elemental composition that reflects the primary constituents of the cobalt-chromium (Co–Cr) implant alloy, which includes cobalt (Co), chromium (Cr), nickel (Ni), and molybdenum (Mo). Notably, the surface of the EDM-treated sample exhibited additional elements, specifically oxygen and carbon, alongside the base alloy components. This observation indicates that the elevated temperatures reached during the EDM process likely facilitated chemical interactions between the molten alloy and the dielectric fluid, typically water. Such interactions can lead to the formation of oxide layers on the material surface, thereby modifying its surface chemistry and characteristics. The presence of these oxide formations is further verified by the XRD pattern presented in Fig. 7.9c. The identified oxides, which include chromium oxide (Cr_2O_3), silicon oxide (SiO_2), beryllium oxide (BeO), and phosphorus nitride (P_3N_5), are well-documented for their potential to enhance the biocompatibility of implant surfaces. This enhancement is particularly crucial in biomedical applications, where material compatibility with biological tissues is essential for successful implantation and long-term functionality. Additionally, the analysis revealed the presence of carbides such as chromium carbide (Cr_7C_3) and tungsten carbide (WC) on the surface of the EDM-modified sample. These carbides play a significant role in increasing the surface hardness of the implant [9, 10]. The improvement in surface hardness is critical, as it directly correlates with enhanced wear resistance, which is vital for the longevity and performance of the implant in a physiological environment [11, 12]. Therefore, the modifications introduced through the EDM process not only improve the biocompatibility of the Co–Cr alloy but also significantly increase its durability against wear and tear during use.

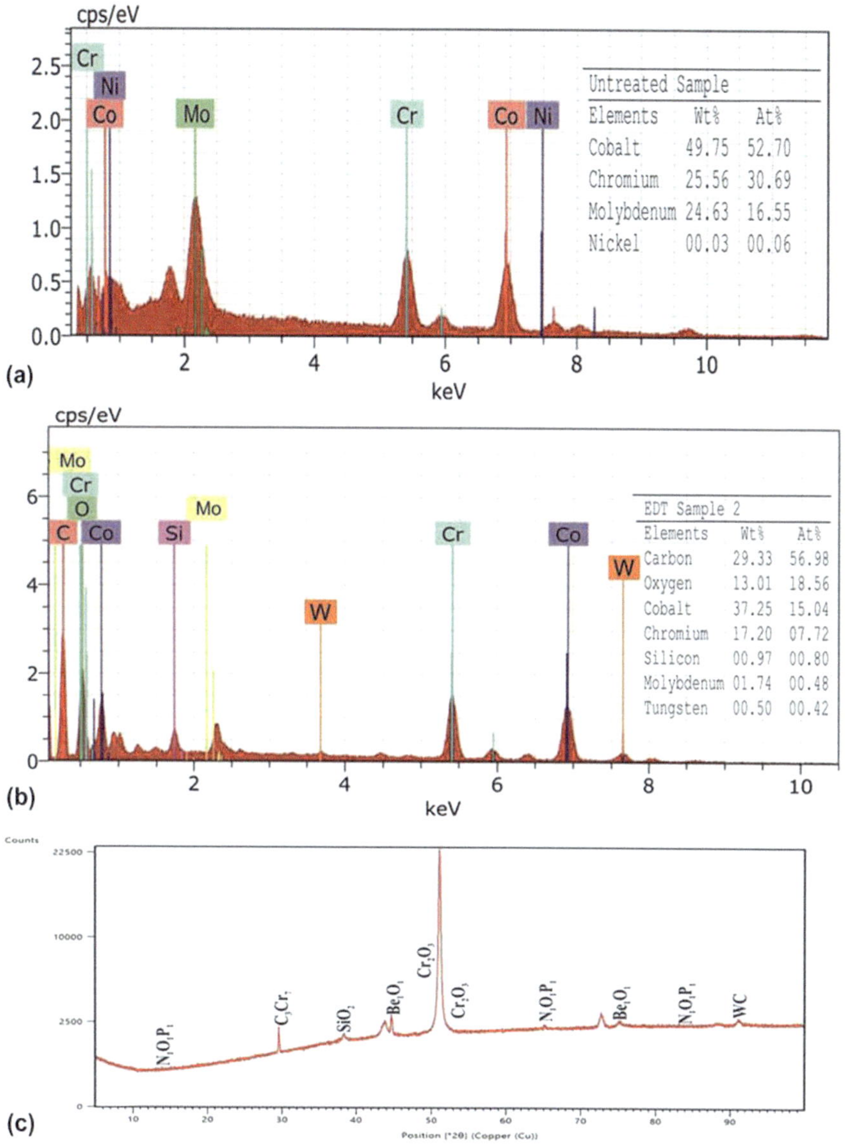

Fig. 7.9 EDS elemental spectrum of **a** untreated and **b** EDT Sample 2; **c** XRD pattern of EDT Sample 2. Reproduced with permission from Springer Nature [1]

7.3 Discussion

The primary objective of this investigation was to comprehensively assess the cytocompatibility and tribological performance of cobalt-chromium (Co–Cr) implant alloys that were subjected to electrical discharge treatment (EDT). This method involves using electrical discharges to create surface modifications that could enhance the properties of the material. To determine cell viability, we utilized an MTT assay, a colorimetric assay that measures cellular metabolic activity as an indicator of cell health and viability. This assay was conducted on both untreated specimens and those that underwent EDT. Among all the samples tested, Sample 2 stood out as the most promising. It was processed using specific parameters: a discharge current of 10 A, a pulse-on time of 200 μs, a pulse-off time of 60 μs, and a W–Cu electrode immersed in deionized water. This configuration resulted in the highest observed cell viability, approximately 88%. Microscopic examination revealed that a significant number of viable cells were visibly adhered to the surface of Sample 2, indicating its strong biocompatibility. In addition to cytocompatibility, we also evaluated the tribological behavior of the samples, which is crucial for understanding how materials perform under frictional conditions. Sample 2 exhibited exceptional tribological performance, characterized by a low wear rate of approximately 1.2×10^{-7} mm^3/Nm, equivalent to about 0.02 mm^3 of material loss, and a coefficient of friction of 0.29. These results suggest that Sample 2 can endure wear more effectively than its untreated counterparts. The observed improvement in wear characteristics is primarily attributed to the formation of surface oxides and carbides during the EDT process. These surface modifications not only enhanced the material's hardness by 1.75 times compared to the untreated substrate but also contributed to its biocompatibility, making it a compelling candidate for biomedical applications.

Furthermore, the results from this Stage III study were carefully compared with findings from previous investigations. During Stage I, Co–Cr samples were machined using a graphite electrode under full factorial experimental conditions. This earlier study identified the optimal spark energy range necessary for effective treatment. Cytocompatibility in that phase was quantified using the MCF-7 (Michigan Cancer Foundation-7) human adenocarcinoma cell line, where the best-performing sample achieved around 80% cell viability. Together, these findings contribute to a deeper understanding of how EDT can enhance the performance and compatibility of Co–Cr implant alloys in medical applications.

Research conducted by Qin et al. [13] provided significant insights into the effects of chitosan coatings on Co–Cr–Mo alloys. Their findings indicated that such coatings could enhance the viability of MC3T3-E1 cells to approximately 82%. Additionally, the wear resistance of these alloys was notably improved, exhibiting a minimal wear rate of 1.1×10^{-7} mm^3/Nm. This outcome aligns closely with the results observed in the current study, highlighting the effectiveness of chitosan as a surface treatment. In contrast, the work of Alvarez-Vera et al. [14] explored the incorporation of boron into Co–Cr alloys, finding that this modification resulted in wear rates that ranged from 0.05 to 0.10 mm^3. This range indicates a relatively higher wear performance compared to the chitosan-coated alloys. Similarly, Ortega-Saenz et al. [15] documented a volumetric wear rate of 0.517 mm^3 for Co–Cr–Mo alloys subjected to plasma nitriding and Physical Vapor Deposition (PVD) coatings, illustrating the variety of methods available to enhance the wear characteristics of these materials. Further research by Dittrick et al. [16] employed the Laser Engineered Net Shaping Technology (LENSTM) on Co–Cr–Mo alloys, reporting a wear rate of 4×10^{-6} mm^3/Nm. This variation in wear rates across different studies suggests that different processing techniques and material compositions can significantly influence the tribological properties of Co–Cr alloys.

Overall, the findings from this Stage III analysis confirm that the EDT-processed Co–Cr alloy, particularly Sample 2, demonstrated remarkable improvements in both cytocompatibility and wear resistance. The development of tribochemical surfaces, enriched with layers of oxides, nitrides, phosphides, and carbides, played a crucial role in enhancing the alloy's bioactivity and its resistance to mechanical degradation. Importantly, the optimal surface treatment parameters included a 10 A current with a 60 μs pulse-on time and a 150 μs pause time. These specific conditions were identified as yielding the best results concerning biocompatibility and tribological performance, ensuring that the material could withstand the rigors of its intended medical applications. Additionally, Stage II results highlighted that these surface modifications not only improved wear resistance but also enhanced corrosion resistance and hemocompatibility. This emphasizes the considerable potential of thermoelectric surface treatments for Co–Cr implants, suggesting a promising avenue for future research and development in biomaterials engineering.

7.4 Conclusions

The surface of a biomedical-grade cobalt-chromium (Co–Cr) alloy was systematically modified using EDM to assess its biological compatibility and tribological properties, which are critical for its application in medical implants. This study involved a comparative analysis between the EDM-treated samples and untreated control samples to evaluate the enhancements brought about by the surface modification. The in-vitro cytotoxicity assessment revealed that the EDM-treated samples exhibited notably improved biocompatibility. Particularly, MG-63 osteoblast-like cell viability was significantly higher in the machined samples compared to the untreated counterparts, indicating that the EDM process not only altered the surface characteristics but also positively influenced cellular interactions, which are essential for the performance of orthopedic implants. Furthermore, the tribological evaluation demonstrated that the treated surfaces had enhanced wear resistance and reduced friction, factors that are crucial in minimizing wear and prolonging the lifespan of implants within the body. The friction and wear tests indicated substantial improvements in the longevity and reliability of the surface, aligning with the mechanical demands of orthopedic applications. To elucidate the underlying mechanisms driving these improvements, advanced analytical techniques such as X-ray Diffraction and

Energy Dispersive X-ray Spectroscopy were employed. These analyses confirmed the formation of beneficial oxide and carbide phases on the surface of the alloy, which are believed to contribute significantly to both the improved biocompatibility and mechanical strength of the material. The research further determined that the optimal processing parameters for EDM treatment included a current setting of 10 A, a pulse on-time of 60 μs, and a pause time of 150 μs. These specific parameters were found to produce the most advantageous surface characteristics and biological responses. In conclusion, the findings of this study suggest that EDM-treated Co–Cr alloys possess considerable potential for use in orthopedic implant applications, offering enhanced biocompatibility, reduced wear, and improved mechanical performance, thereby potentially increasing the success rates of such medical devices.

References

1. Mahajan A, Sidhu SS (2019) Potential of electrical discharge treatment to enhance the in vitro cytocompatibility and tribological performance of Co–Cr implant. J Mater Res 34(16):2837–2847
2. Mahajan A, Sidhu SS, Ablyaz T (2019) EDM surface treatment: an enhanced biocompatible interface. In: Biomaterials in orthopaedics and bone regeneration: design and synthesis. Singapore, pp 33–40
3. Lamichhane Y, Singh G, Bhui AS, Mukhiya P, Kumar P, Thapa B (2019) Surface modification of 316L SS with HAp nano-particles using PMEDM for enhanced biocompatibility. Mater Today Proc 15:336–343
4. Singh B, Singh G, Sidhu BS (2019) Investigation of the in vitro corrosion behavior and biocompatibility of niobium (Nb)-reinforced hydroxyapatite (HA) coating on CoCr alloy for medical implants. J Mater Res 34(10):1678–1691
5. Mahajan A, Devgan S, Kalyanasundaram D (2022) Electrical discharge machining—a futuristic technique for surface engineering of biomedical alloys: a concise review. Surf Topogr Metrol Prop 10(4):043001
6. Lee WF, Yang TS, Wu YC, Peng PW (2013) Nanoporous biocompatible layer on Ti–6Al–4V alloys enhanced osteoblast-like cell response. J Exp Clin Med 5(3):92–96
7. Ikeuchi K, Morita Y, Yoshida H, Kusaka J (2001) Effect of tribochemical reaction on wear of silicon carbide for joint prostheses. J Ceram Process Res 2:35–37
8. Hesketh J, Ward M, Dowson D, Neville A (2014) The composition of tribofilms produced on metal-on-metal hip bearings. Biomaterials 35:2113–2119
9. Jenko M, Gorensek M, Godec M, Hodnik M, Batic BS, Donik C, Grant JT, Dolinar D (2018) Surface chemistry and microstructure of metallic biomaterials for hip and knee endoprostheses. Appl Surf Sci 427:584–593
10. Im BM, Akiyama E, Habazaki H, Kawashima A, Asami K, Hashimoto K (1995) The effect of phosphorus addition on the corrosion behavior of amorphous Fe-8Cr-P alloys in 9M H_2SO_4. Corros Sci 37(5):709–722
11. Wu P, Zhou CZ, Tang XN (2003) Microstructural characterization and wear behavior of laser cladded nickel-based and tungsten carbide composite coatings. Surf Coat Technol 166(1):84–88
12. Weng Z, Wang A, Wu X, Wang Y, Yang Z (2016) Wear resistance of diode laser-clad Ni/WC composite coatings at different temperatures. Surf Coat Technol 304:283–292
13. Qin L, Feng X, Hafezi M, Zhang Y, Guo J, Dong G, Qin Y (2018) Investigating the tribological and biological performance of covalently grafted chitosan coatings on Co–Cr–Mo alloy. Tribol Int 127:302–312

14. Alvarez-Vera M, Juarez-Hernandez A, Gonzalez-Rivera CE, Mercado-Solis RD, Hernandez-Rodriguez MAL (2013) Biotribological response of Co–Cr alloy with added boron under ball-on-disc tests. Wear 301(1–2):243–249
15. Ortega-Saenz JA, Hernandez-Rodriguez MAL, Ventura-Sobrevilla V, Michalczewski R, Smolik J, Szczerek M (2011) Tribological and corrosion testing of surface engineered surgical grade CoCrMo alloy. Wear 271(9–10):2125–2131
16. Dittrick S, Balla VK, Davies NM, Bose S, Bandyopadhyay A (2011) In-vitro wear rate and Co ion release of compositionally and structurally graded CoCrMo-Ti6Al4V structure. Mater Sci Eng C 31(4):809–814

Chapter 8
Conclusions and Future Scope

This monograph has presented a comprehensive exploration into the surface modification of cobalt-chromium (Co–Cr) alloy using EDM techniques for orthopedic implant applications. The work has systematically addressed the need for improved bioactivity, wear resistance, corrosion resistance, and biocompatibility of Co–Cr implants by developing a novel approach for surface coating with biomaterials. The introductory chapters offered an in-depth overview of the material challenges in orthopedic implants and provided a rationale for choosing Co–Cr alloy, given its excellent mechanical strength, corrosion resistance, and wear properties. However, the inherent bioinert nature of Co–Cr alloy often necessitates surface modifications to enhance its biological response when implanted in the human body. The literature review further highlighted the limitations of existing surface modification techniques and emphasized the potential of EDM as a hybrid process capable of both machining and surface functionalization.

Subsequent chapters detailed the methodology for EDM-based coating using biocompatible powders, particularly titanium and its oxides, as dielectric additives or electrode materials. The process parameters were optimized to achieve desirable surface textures and deposition characteristics. Surface characterization was performed using SEM, EDS, and XRD to confirm the formation of bioactive phases and modified surface layers. The enhanced performance of the modified surfaces was validated through corrosion resistance testing in simulated body fluid, tribological analysis to assess wear resistance, and mechanical integrity evaluation of the coatings. Furthermore, the biocompatibility of the coated surfaces was evaluated through in-vitro cytotoxicity and hemolysis tests. The results indicated that the EDM-modified Co–Cr surfaces not only improved the mechanical and chemical stability of the material but also showed promising bioactivity, making them suitable for long-term orthopedic applications.

© The Author(s), under exclusive license to Springer Nature Singapore Pte Ltd. 2026

A. Mahajan et al., *Surface Modification of Co–Cr Alloy for Orthopaedic Applications*,
Biomedical Materials for Multi-functional Applications,
https://doi.org/10.1007/978-981-95-4029-7_8

8.1 Summary of Key Findings

Cobalt-chromium (Co–Cr) alloys have become widely used materials in orthopedic applications, primarily due to their superior mechanical properties, impressive corrosion resistance, and strong biocompatibility, which makes them suitable for use in medical implants [1–3]. However, as the demand for enhanced performance in orthopedic devices grows, it has become important to improve their surface properties. Improving the surface properties can significantly impact their biological integration with human tissues and their resistance to wear over time. To address these challenges, a range of surface engineering techniques has been explored, including CVD, PVD, laser texturing, ion implantation, plasma spraying, and the application of bioactive coatings. Each of these methods has demonstrated potential benefits in optimizing both the wear characteristics (tribological properties) and the biological interaction of the materials with surrounding tissues. Despite the promising developments associated with these surface treatments, there remain significant concerns regarding the long-term reliability of these modifications. Issues related to the scalability of the manufacturing processes and cost-effectiveness also pose challenges for widespread clinical application. In the current study, we investigated the effects of EDM on medical-grade Co–Cr alloy specimens. The EDM process was found to create modified surfaces featuring porous metallic residues that closely mimic the architecture of natural bone microstructures. This resemblance suggests a potential for improved compatibility with human biological systems, which could enhance osseointegration and overall implant performance. By fine-tuning the composition of the tool electrodes used in EDM and optimizing the machining parameters, we were able to achieve notable improvements in the biofunctional performance of the treated alloys. These refinements indicate that EDM may serve as a viable and efficient surface modification technique for orthopedic applications, potentially leading to better patient outcomes and increased longevity of implants [4–6].

Stage I

This phase of the study focused on analyzing the effect of EDM parameters on the surface morphology of cobalt-chromium (Co–Cr) implants, as well as evaluating their subsequent biological response through a series of in-vitro experiments. A full factorial design was implemented to systematically investigate how different levels of spark energy influenced various surface characteristics.

- The results indicated that surfaces treated with spark energies between 960 and 1500 J exhibited enhanced micro- and macro-scale roughness. This specific roughness is believed to facilitate improved cell adhesion and proliferation, creating a more favorable environment for cell growth [7].
- Furthermore, the EDM-modified samples demonstrated significantly increased cell viability for both MCF-7 (human breast cancer) and HeLa (cervical cancer) cells. Additionally, these samples showed a favorable hemolytic activity profile, exhibiting lower rates of hemolysis compared to untreated control samples, indicating reduced toxicity and better compatibility with blood components.

- Notably, Trial 8, which utilized a current of 5 A and a pulse on-time of 200 μs, yielded surfaces that were rich in phosphides. These surfaces displayed exceptional cytocompatibility and hemocompatibility, making them particularly promising for medical applications in implantology.
- Overall, the EDM process not only facilitates the precise removal of material but also enables the creation of functional surface textures. This capability is crucial for enhancing the clinical viability of Co–Cr implants, as it significantly increases design precision and optimizes the implants' interaction with biological tissues [8, 9].

Stage II

This stage of the research focused on investigating various electrode materials, graphite, tungsten, and tungsten-copper (W–Cu), to determine how these materials influence the machining outcomes. To systematically evaluate the impacts of different machining parameters, an L18 orthogonal array design was implemented. This design allowed for a thorough assessment of how factors such as electrical current, pulse duration, electrode material, and the dielectric medium affect both corrosion resistance and biological responses. The key findings from the investigation include the following:

- The treated surfaces exhibited significant improvements in corrosion resistance, an essential quality for materials used in medical implants. Additionally, the surfaces maintained compatibility with blood, which is crucial for any material that comes into contact with biological tissues.
- Among the different electrode materials tested, the tungsten-copper (W–Cu) electrode was found to be particularly effective. It generated a highly corrosion-resistant surface when used under conditions of high pulse-on-time combined with minimal pause duration, indicating its suitability for creating durable and reliable implant surfaces.
- Detailed analysis of the surface characteristics revealed that the machining process led to the formation of various compounds, including carbides, oxides, and borides. These compounds played a significant role in enhancing both the corrosion resistance of the surfaces and their biological activity, likely improving the interface between the implant and the surrounding biological tissues [10, 11].
- ANOVA was conducted to identify the most effective parameters for machining. The results indicated that the optimal conditions consisted of a current of 10 A, a pulse on-time of 200 μs, and a pause time of 60 μs, with the machining process occurring in deionized water using the W–Cu electrode.
- Overall, this study highlights the potential of EDM as a viable method for enhancing the performance of Co–Cr alloy surfaces, making them more suitable for biomedical applications.

Stage III

In this phase of our research, we conducted an in-depth investigation into the effectiveness of EDM in enhancing both the biological and mechanical performance of materials, particularly focusing on cobalt-chromium (Co–Cr) implants. The treatment process employed a tungsten-copper (W–Cu) electrode within a controlled deionized water environment, which is known to minimize contamination and maximize the accuracy of the EDM process. Following the treatment, we rigorously assessed the surface properties of the samples using various analytical techniques aimed at evaluating their biocompatibility and tribological behavior.

- Cytotoxicity assays were performed using MG-63 osteoblast cells, a widely recognized model for studying bone-related cellular responses. The results demonstrated that these cells exhibited significantly higher viability on the EDM-treated samples compared to those that were left untreated, suggesting that the EDM process not only enhanced the surface characteristics of the implants but also made them more favorable for biological interaction.
- Furthermore, we evaluated the tribological performance of the modified samples. The data revealed a notable reduction in wear rates and lower friction coefficients when compared to untreated samples, indicating improved durability and wear resistance, crucial factors for orthopedic applications where implants undergo constant mechanical stress.
- To complement these findings, XRD and EDX analyses. These analyses confirmed the formation of hard carbide and oxide layers on the surface of the EDM-treated samples, which are believed to be responsible for enhanced surface performance. The formation of these layers, which are indicative of oxidation and carbide strengthening, plays a significant role in protecting the underlying material and improving its longevity under mechanical loads.
- Through extensive experimentation, we identified the optimal EDM processing conditions: a current of 10 A, a pulse on-time of 60 μs, and a pause time of 150 μs. These parameters resulted in surfaces exhibiting superior biological compatibility and tribological characteristics, making them particularly suitable for orthopedic applications where both bone integration and mechanical robustness are critical [12, 13].
- In conclusion, our findings strongly position EDM-treated Co–Cr implants as highly promising candidates for use in orthopedic procedures, offering not only enhanced mechanical performance but also improved biocompatibility, which is essential for the long-term success of orthopedic implants in patients [14, 15].

8.2 Future Research Directions

Surface engineering through unconventional methods, particularly EDM, represents an exciting and rapidly evolving frontier in the field of biomaterials science. This study provides strong evidence that EDM is a viable and effective tool for enhancing the surface properties of cobalt-chromium (Co–Cr) alloys, which are commonly used in various medical implants. However, several critical areas warrant further investigation to fully understand and optimize the benefits of this technique:

- Conducting a thorough analysis of post-machining residual stress is essential, as it affects the long-term performance and durability of the treated materials. Additionally, assessing surface energy, microhardness, and wettability can yield valuable insights into the interactions of the alloy surface with biological environments, which are important for improving biocompatibility.
- Implementing powder-mixed EDM could enhance the surface characteristics by integrating conductive and abrasive powders into the EDM process. This approach may lead to improved corrosion resistance and better biological performance, thereby increasing the lifespan and effectiveness of implants.
- Future research should prioritize in-vivo experiments to evaluate real-time clinical effectiveness and to understand how the enhanced surface properties of EDM-treated implants interact with biological tissues in a living organism. Such studies are vital for translating laboratory findings into practical clinical applications.
- Exploring hybrid machining techniques that combine EDM with complementary methods, such as laser machining or ultrasonic machining, could optimize the surface functionality of implants. These hybrid approaches may provide synergistic benefits, leading to superior outcomes such as improved mechanical properties and enhanced surface texture.
- It is also important to conduct comprehensive biocompatibility assessments, including implantation studies, irritation tests, and sensitization evaluations. These tests are essential for demonstrating the safety and efficacy of the modified materials and will be critical in supporting regulatory certification and acceptance.
- Finally, extending this surface modification strategy to other widely used implantable metals, such as stainless steel or titanium alloys, has significant implications. Such an expansion could broaden the clinical applicability of EDM techniques, thereby addressing a wider range of medical needs and improving patient outcomes across various fields of implant dentistry, orthopedics, and cardiovascular devices. By addressing these areas of exploration, future research can significantly contribute to the advancement of biomaterials science and the quality of medical implants used in clinical settings.

In conclusion, this work establishes a technically viable and biologically acceptable pathway for enhancing the surface performance of Co–Cr alloys, pushing the boundaries for their safe and long-term use in orthopedic implants. EDM allows precise deposition of bioactive materials, resulting in improved osseointegration, enhanced corrosion and wear resistance, and overall better implant-host interaction. This monograph serves as a reference for researchers, material scientists, and biomedical engineers striving to enhance the surface functionality and longevity of metallic implants for orthopedic applications. By advancing the scientific understanding of surface modification techniques for Co–Cr alloys, the work not only addresses current challenges in implant technology but also lays the foundation for future interdisciplinary collaborations. Bridging materials science, biomedical engineering, and clinical research, the findings presented here aim to improve patient outcomes through the development of more effective and biocompatible implant surfaces.

References

1. Saini M, Singh Y, Arora P, Arora V, Jain K (2015) Implant biomaterials: a comprehensive review. World J Clin Cases 3:52
2. Devgan S, Mahajan A, Mahajan V (2023) Machining performance of cobalt-chromium and β-type titanium biomedical alloy. In: Materials for biomedical simulation: design, development and characterization. Springer Nature Singapore, Singapore, pp 85–91
3. Mantrala KM, Das M, Balla VK, Rao CS, Rao VK (2014) Laser-deposited CoCrMo alloy: microstructure, wear, and electrochemical properties. J Mater Res 29:2021–2027
4. Tarzia V, Bottio T, Testolin L, Gerosa G (2007) Extended (31 years) durability of Starr–Edwards prosthesis in mitral position. Interact Cardiovasc Thorac Surg 6:570–571
5. Mahajan A, Sidhu SS, Ablyaz T (2019) EDM surface treatment: an enhanced biocompatible interface. In: Biomaterials in orthopaedics and bone regeneration: design and synthesis. Springer Singapore, Singapore, pp 33–40
6. Bhaumik M, Maity K (2019) Effect of electrode materials on different EDM aspects of titanium alloy. Silicon 11(1):187–196
7. Singh G, Sidhu SS, Bains PS, Singh M, Bhui AS (2020) On surface modification of Ti alloy by electro discharge coating using hydroxyapatite powder mixed dielectric with graphite tool. J Bio- Tribo-Corros 6(3):91
8. Mahajan A, Sidhu SS (2018) Enhancing biocompatibility of Co–Cr alloy implants via electrical discharge process. Mater Technol 33(8):524–531
9. Singh G, Ablyaz TR, Shlykov ES, Muratov KR, Bhui AS, Sidhu SS (2020) Enhancing corrosion and wear resistance of Ti6Al4V alloy using CNTs mixed electro-discharge process. Micromachines 11(9):850
10. Al-Amin M, Abdul-Rani AM, Danish M, Rubaiee S, Mahfouz AB, Thompson HM et al (2021) Investigation of coatings, corrosion and wear characteristics of machined biomaterials through hydroxyapatite mixed-EDM process: a review. Materials 14(13):3597
11. Mahajan A, Sidhu SS (2019) In vitro corrosion and hemocompatibility evaluation of electrical discharge treated cobalt–chromium implant. J Mater Res 34(8):1363–1370
12. Li G, Wang L, Pan W, Yang F, Jiang W, Wu X, Kong X, Dai K, Hao Y (2016) In vitro and in vivo study of additive manufactured porous Ti6Al4V scaffolds for repairing bone defects. Sci Rep 6:34072
13. Mahajan A, Sidhu SS (2019) Potential of electrical discharge treatment to enhance the in vitro cytocompatibility and tribological performance of Co–Cr implant. J Mater Res 34(16):2837–2847
14. Tuna SH, Pekmez NO, Kurkçuoglu I (2015) Corrosion resistance assessment of Co–Cr alloy frameworks fabricated by CAD/CAM milling, laser sintering, and casting methods. J Prosthet Dent 114(5):725–734
15. Qiu J, Yu WQ, Zhang FQ, Smales RJ, Zhang YL, Lu CH (2011) Corrosion behaviour and surface analysis of a Co–Cr and two Ni–Cr dental alloys before and after simulated porcelain firing. Eur J Oral Sci 119(1):93–101

MIX
Papier aus verantwortungsvollen Quellen
Paper from responsible sources
FSC® C105338

If you have any concerns about our products,
you can contact us on
ProductSafety@springernature.com

In case Publisher is established outside the EU,
the EU authorized representative is:
Springer Nature Customer Service Center GmbH
Europaplatz 3, 69115 Heidelberg, Germany

Printed by Libri Plureos GmbH
in Hamburg, Germany